Shared Care for

Rheumatology

Shared Care for
Rheumatology

Gillian Hosie MB, ChB, DA
General Practitioner
Knightswood Medical Practice
Glasgow, UK

Max Field BSc, MD, FRCP
Consultant and Senior Lecturer in Rheumatology
Centre for Rheumatic Diseases
University of Glasgow
Glasgow, UK

with additional material by
Mharie Brandon
Senior Physiotherapist
Glasgow Royal Infirmary
Glasgow, UK

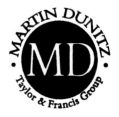

© 2002 Martin Dunitz Ltd, a member of the Taylor & Francis group

First published in the United Kingdom in 2002
by Martin Dunitz Ltd, The Livery House, 7–9 Pratt Street, London NW1 0AE

Tel.:   +44 (0) 20 74822202
Fax.:   +44 (0) 20 72670159
E-mail: info@dunitz.co.uk
Website: http://www.dunitz.co.uk

Although every effort has been made to ensure that all owners of copyright material have been acknowledged in this publication, we would be glad to acknowledge in subsequent reprints or editions any omissions brought to our attention.

The Authors have asserted their right under the Copyright, Designs and Patents Act 1988 to be identified as the Authors of this Work.

Although every effort has been made to ensure that drug doses and other information are presented accurately in this publication, the ultimate responsibility rests with the prescribing physician. Neither the publishers nor the authors can be held responsible for errors or for any consequences arising from the use of information contained herein. For detailed prescribing information or instructions on the use of any product or procedure discussed herein, please consult the prescribing information or instructional material issued by the manufacturer.

A CIP record for this book is available from the British Library.

ISBN 1-901865-10-X

Distributed in the USA by	Distributed in Canada by	Distributed in the rest of the world by
Fulfilment Center	Taylor & Francis	ITPS Limited
Taylor & Francis	74 Rolark Drive	Cheriton House
7625 Empire Drive	Scarborough, Ontario M1R 4G2,	North Way,Andover, Hampshire
Florence, KY 41042, USA	Canada	SP10 5BE, UK
Toll Free Tel.: +1 800 634 7064	Toll Free Tel.: +1 877 226 2237	Tel.: +44 (0)1264 332424
E-mail: cserve@routledge_ny.com	E-mail: tal_fran@istar.ca	E-mail: reception@itps.co.uk

Composition from the authors' electronic files by John Saunders Design & Production
Printed and bound in Spain by E.G. Zure

Foreword

Rheumatology is a discipline which encompasses a broad range of conditions which result in pain, stiffness and loss of function. Those involved in the professional care of patients presenting with musculoskeletal disorders must be able to work in a team involving individuals working in both primary and secondary care. Patients with musculoskeletal pain need to be managed effectively in the primary sector but also should be referred appropriately for specialist care when the diagnosis is in doubt or when management is problematic.

This new text book uniquely brings together a general practitioner and a rheumatologist who have developed a combined approach to the diagnosis and management of musculoskeletal conditions. Dr. Gill Hosie and Dr. Max Field are both highly skilled in this area and they have produced a practical handbook which will be very helpful to all healthcare professionals working in the field of rheumatology. I am very happy to commend this very useful introduction to common musculoskeletal problems.

R.D. STURROCK
Past President British Society for Rheumatology
Currently Chair of the Board of Trustees of
the Arthritis Research Campaign

Contents

Acknowledgements

We are most grateful for the support that we have had during the writing of this text. Firstly, secretarial assistance has been made available through the Arthritis Research Campaign ICAC grant No S0590, and we are grateful for their financial support and to Mrs Carol Ryder for her continued help in this area. We are also grateful to Mrs Isobel Douglas of the Knightswood Medical Practice for secretarial input.

Line drawings were undertaken by Stephen Timpson, and we are indebted to him for his giving up his vacation to produce these excellent figures. We would also like to acknowledge that some pictures have been donated by Professors R.D. Sturrock and P.J. Venables, Drs. I.B. McInnes, H. Capell, D. Kane, A. Forrester, R. McKenzie and Messers I.B. Kelley. J. Field, R. Simpson, and R. Duncan without whose assistance this book would not have been illustrated as well as has been possible. We also acknowledge assistance and support from the Primary Care Rheumatology Society and from the University of Bath Diploma in Primary Care Rheumatology who have allowed us to reproduce Figure 23.3 from Module 5 of the Distance Learning course.

Editorial assistance been supplied by Jonathon Gregory, John Saunders and Pete Stevenson who have demonstrated remarkable composure during the production of the written text.

Finally we would like to express our thanks to our respective spouses who have been very patient and uncomplaining during the last twelve months for which we are extremely grateful.

chapter 1

Introduction

Musculo-skeletal problems are very common within the community and make up around 15% of a general practitioner's workload. There are also many people with joint pain who do not present to primary care: they consider muscle and joint pain to be a normal part of life, and particularly in the older age groups, an inevitable part of the ageing process and something which they must just endure. Therefore, the burden of disease within the community may be considerably greater than we think.

Education in the management of rheumatological problems is variable and many primary care physicians have very little training and expertise in managing these conditions.

In rheumatology, as in many areas of medicine, some conditions are common and can and should be managed almost entirely within primary care, whilst other conditions are rarer and more complex and require management by experts in rheumatology within secondary care. Inevitably there will be an overlap. Patients and their conditions do not fit into neat categories and providers of both primary and secondary care must be prepared to work together to produce the best outcome for patients—a true shared care approach.

Even when patients with complex problems are referred to and managed within secondary care, the primary care physician in the United Kingdom is still responsible for dealing with the patient's other medical problems and for prescribing drugs. The responsibility for drug prescription lies with the doctor who writes the prescription —the primary care physician. He or she, therefore, must be aware of the mode of action, potential side effects and interactions of drugs used in secondary care and be prepared to be involved in monitoring patients taking some of these medications.

Many musculo-skeletal conditions can be improved by patient education and advice and in chronic painful joint problems the long-term support of a medical team, whether in primary or secondary care, can be invaluable. This kind of education and support, however, can only be provided by those confident in and knowledgeable about the disease area. This book is not intended to be a comprehensive textbook of rheumatology but rather a practical handbook to aid management within primary care.

The first part of the book looks at basic skills relevant to the management of musculo-skeletal problems including history, examination and investigations. In the second part there is a description of a number of common and important conditions and in the third part we look at some specific problems as they may present to the general practitioner. Finally, we discuss options for management including patient education and self-management, physical therapy, pharmacological therapy and surgery.

Part 1

BASIC SKILLS

chapter 2

Assessment of the musculo-skeletal system

THE EXTENT OF THE PROBLEM

Musculo-skeletal diseases make up 15% of the primary care physician's workload every year. Calculating an average list of 2,500 per general practitioner this represents 375 consultations each year. Over 20,000,000 people have some complaint affecting the musculo-skeletal system each year in the United Kingdom, with a total cost of musculo-skeletal disease to the National Health Service estimated at 8% of the budget.

Many of these disorders are peri-articular, and despite not involving the joint itself, present with pain as the predominant symptom, often erroneously attributed to the joints. Most are self-limiting, resolving with simple analgesia but physiotherapy may be required. However, it is imperative to identify inflammatory synovitis because active early treatment by a multidisciplinary team improves symptom control and reduces joint damage.

The common disorders of the musculo-skeletal system are delineated in Figure 2.1. The soft tissue diseases and back pain are the most prevalent. Osteoarthritis is common in Western populations with the changes in demography in the first world, and is the commonest cause of joint replacement. Inflammatory arthropathies, while making up a minority of the total, produce protracted forms of disease which also result in total joint destruction.

Before going into detail about the history and examination of the musculo-skeletal system it might be beneficial to describe the components thereof.

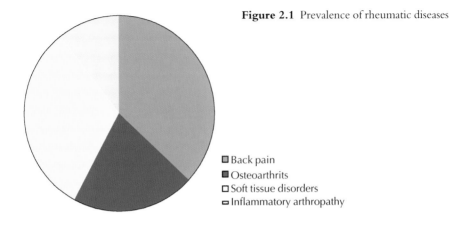

Figure 2.1 Prevalence of rheumatic diseases

☐ Back pain
■ Osteoarthrits
☐ Soft tissue disorders
▫ Inflammatory arthropathy

CONSTITUENT COMPONENTS OF THE MUSCULO-SKELETAL SYSTEM

Bone

Apart from forming the major reservoir for calcium and phosphate in the body, the bones also form the support component for the musculo-skeletal system. Within the long bones (femur, radius etc.) there are two distinct bone forms with differing functions. Collagen type 1 predominates in both, forming multiple cross-links with other bone proteins to provide the necessary tensile strength. These proteins are manufactured by osteoblasts during bone development, and calcium in the form of hydroxyapatite is subsequently deposited between the fibrils to provide mechanical rigidity. During life, bone synthesis goes hand in hand with bone degradation. Osteoclasts destroy bone tissue releasing calcium from this store and allowing constant remodelling of each bone dependent on the mechanical stresses imposed upon them.

Cortical bone forms the major supporting function, and is found over the whole bone surface, but is thicker and stronger in the bone shaft. Histologically cortical bone consists of a tightly packed dense structure of Haversian canals with central arterial and venous supply (Figure 2.2). These run vertically along the bone parallel to its surface providing a tubular structure supporting the body weight through its vertical axis. However, cortical bone has little strength when stress is applied in the horizontal plane. By comparison, cancellous or trabecular bone exists predominantly within the ends of the long bones. As the collagen fibrils are not parallel to the surface

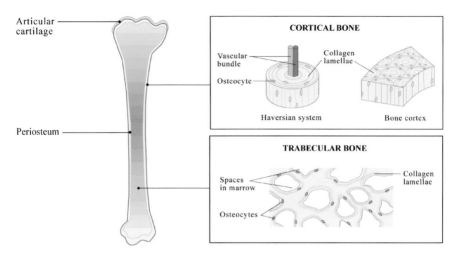

Figure 2.2 *Bone structure*

(see Figure 2.2), trabecular bone provides support by virtue of its scaffolding structure within the thinner cortical bone at sites where horizontal stress is exerted like the femoral neck and the lower end of the radius and ulna.

The synovial joint

The synovial joint allows controlled movement within the rigid skeletal structure, but this flexibility is limited for each joint by the peri-articular structures (Figure 2.3).

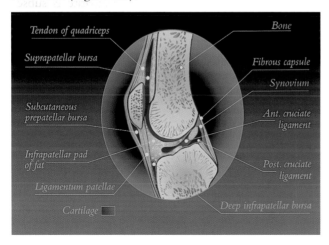

Figure 2.3 *Synovial joint pathology*

Cartilage

Articular (hyaline) cartilage surround the epiphyses of the long bones lining their articulating surface. Cartilage provides a structure with some resistance to compression exerted as the two surfaces come in contact during movement. It consists of a semi-rigid collagen (types II, IV and VI) matrix made by chondrocytes that provide the tensile strength. The other major constituent is proteoglycans that consist of a protein core to which are linked carbohydrate chains. Proteoglycans retain water, that can be extruded under pressure, providing an elasticity to cartilage that allows reversible changes of shape to occur as the two surfaces oppose one another, and providing resistance to compression.

Synovial fluid

The fluid within the normal synovial joint is an aqueous exudate from serum with similar concentrations of ions but lower glucose levels. Synovial fluid provides nutrients for the avascular cartilage during joint inactivity, but it also provides lubrication during joint movement. The most abundant components covering this action are the glycoproteins hyaluronan and lubricin. Synovial fluid is subsequently absorbed into the local lymphatic drainage.

Synovial membrane

The normal membrane lines the structures around the synovial joint including the capsule, intra-articular ligaments, and periarticular tendons and bursae. The membrane is a relatively acellular matrix consisting of resident fibroblasts within a collagen framework. The synovial lining layer consists of type A cells derived from macrophages thought to have a scavenging role, and the type B fibroblast derived cells that are considered responsible for synthesis of the synovial fluid glycoproteins. Synovial membrane lining the tendons and bursae produce fluid locally that facilitates tendon, skin and muscle movement over underlying bony structures.

Ligaments

Ligaments consist of a firm collagen type I framework and provide rigidity, particularly at the extremes of joint movement. They are attached to bone usually close to the articular surface of the joint at the enthesis where the collagen fibres interdigitate with bone collagens. However, as ligaments come into contact with the joint capsule they can be integrated therein providing added strength.

Muscles

Muscles have an overlapping structure of myosin filaments that are linked by phosphate bonds that require energy to be set up. As these bonds are broken the myosin filaments move across one another and the bonds reform. The movement of the myofibrils is translated on a gross scale to muscle contraction enabling the joint to move in a controlled manner. Many muscles change their structure at one end close to the joint to one containing more collagen type I transforming the muscle into a tendon that inserts into bone at separate entheses.

chapter 3

History and examination in the rheumatic diseases

Diagnosis and assessment in patients with rheumatic diseases requires careful history and physical examination. Investigations confirm a diagnosis, but they are rarely specific for any one disease and should be interpreted with caution in the absence of clinical findings.

HISTORY

A good historian will readily establish a diagnosis by characterising the patient's most important symptoms and their effect on lifestyle and family. Although most patients present with pain, stiffness or disability, symptoms in the rheumatic diseases can be a manifestation of more systemic pathology, so thorough detailed enquiry and examination is mandatory.

Two screening questions are useful to establish the relevance of any joint pathology:

- Do you suffer from any pain or stiffness in the arms, legs, neck or back?
- Do you have difficulty with washing and dressing or going up and down stairs?

If the answer is yes to either, then a more detailed history should be obtained (Table 3.1), establishing the site, character, chronicity and impact of symptoms on the patient's lifestyle.

Pain

Pain is generalised in conditions such as fibromyalgia with widespread poorly focussed tenderness over recognised pressure points. Regional pain is often

---

Table 3.1 Useful questions in patients with rheumatic diseases

General questions
- Do you suffer from any pain or stiffness in the arms, legs, neck or back?
- Do you have difficulty with washing and dressing or going up and down stairs?

Specific questions
- Demographic details
- Location and character of joint pain and effect on activities of daily living
- Severity and effect of pain on hobbies, ability to work and home life
- Duration, radiation, temporal characteristics of pain
- Exacerbating/relieving factors, effects of treatment
- Joint swelling, temporal relationships and relation to stiffness
- Systemic features – weight loss, fevers, Raynaud's phenomenon
- Enquiry about other system involvement
- Previous history, drug use, family and social history

---

poorly characterised from tissues of the musculo-skeletal system, but the site can give an indication as to the area for more detailed examination. Pain from the cervical region can radiate to the shoulder and upper arm. Similarly, prolapse of L4/L5 inter-vertebral discs presents with radiating pain to the buttock, lower limb and often to the foot, whilst that from the upper lumbar disc disease goes to the thigh, each with the appropriate neurological deficit. Hip pain can be referred to the knee frequently causing diagnostic confusion, and median nerve entrapment produces pain that radiates both up and down the arm. The character of the pain, such as shooting or throbbing, may give a clue as to a possible neurogenic or infective aetiology.

Timing

Classically, degenerative pain is exacerbated after exercise and at the end of the day. Inflammatory joint pain usually occurs at rest and on use, but characteristically improves during exercise. Severe metastatic bone pain is relentless, persisting throughout the day, interfering with sleep. Exacerbating factors can also provide diagnostic clues. Tenderness over the lateral epicondyle of the humerus (tennis elbow) is worse during forearm supination. The buttock and leg pain of spinal stenosis deteriorates with walking, and is relieved by bending forwards, a process that is thought to relieve pressure on nerve routes. Although the different descriptions of pain in inflammatory and degenerative disease are recognised in textbooks, frequently they overlap causing some confusion to the unprepared.

Stiffness

Stiffness is an important feature in patients with inflammatory synovitis. The arthritis in ankylosing spondylitis, systemic lupus erythematosus and rheumatoid arthritis produces long lasting early morning stiffness, albeit in different joints that respond to appropriate treatment. The stiffness from degenerative disease however, is short lasting, often affecting only one localised weight bearing joint. In either instance initiation of movement after rest is a significant problem.

Impact

Impact of the symptoms is particularly relevant. Musculo–skeletal diseases cause pain and limit the activities of daily living. Enquiry about which activities the patient enjoys but cannot presently undertake, helps to gauge some idea of the patient's expectation in relation to the disease, disability and their handicap. The impact of septic arthritis in the knee is significant loss of function in the affected joint that will have a major impact on a patient with underlying rheumatoid arthritis. However, the degree of increased disability and handicap over and above that already present is unlikely to be as significant as that affecting a young and fit man working for an outward bound school.

Other common symptoms

Specific enquiry should be made into the presence or absence of joint swelling, development of joint deformities, cracking of joints, clicking or locking of joints and loss of movement. Bone swelling and deformity implies a long-standing destructive process whilst the presence of soft tissue painful swelling suggests an acute or sub–acute active synovitis. Locking implies an intra-articular mechanical abnormality such as trapping of soft tissue (cartilage or synovium between the articulating surfaces restricting complete movement). A trigger finger is thought to develop in a similar way with synovial tissue getting trapped as the tendon moves up and down its synovial sheath. Cracking and clicking of joints in young people is usually not significant and is thought to represent changes in surface tension in synovial fluid. These may be significant when involving a demonstrated mechanical abnormality within the joint architecture in degenerative osteoarthritis.

The general enquiry

The general enquiry is particularly significant, as inflammatory arthropathies can frequently be presenting symptoms of other diseases; a comprehensive history covering the skin, eyes, lungs, kidneys, gastrointestinal tract, as well as constitutional symptoms of malaise, weight loss, fevers and night sweats can be informative. A drug history is also helpful for example in cases of gout (thiazide diuretic) and systemic lupus erythematosus (minocycline, hydrallazine). A previous medical history may also identify miscarriages, pleurisy or tuberculosis that could impact on diagnosis and treatment. Similarly, as there is a genetic element to many rheumatic diseases a comprehensive family history can be invaluable.

Psychological problems

Psychological problems can precede development of chronic pain and disability. However, anxiety and depression can occur as a sequelae of underlying symptoms and major psychiatric disturbances can occur as a result of disease process such as systemic lupus erythematosus. Sleep disturbances and lethargy are frequent sequelae of fibromyalgia.

EXAMINATION OF THE MUSCULO-SKELETAL SYSTEM

This can be divided into inspection, palpation and examination of the joint during movement.

Inspection

Inspection of the affected joint should be undertaken at rest and in comparison to the unaffected side (Figure 3.1). Skin should be examined for scars, erythema and rashes, and muscles for atrophy that occurs following disuse in chronic joint disease. Examination of swelling should demonstrate the site and size of any affected lesion and the presence of deformity or asymmetry should be noted. Examination of the joint during movement will demonstrate the range of active movement, the degree of ease with which the joint moves and comparison to the other side will assess the degree of disability. Watching the face during movement will provide a clue as to the presence of pain.

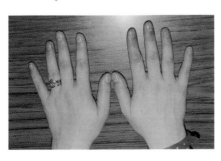

Figure 3.1 *Acute synovitis*

Palpation

Palpation of inflamed joints can be particularly painful. Warmth and tenderness are features of inflammatory joint disease. Close examination may be required to establish the site of pain, such as joint line tenderness in osteoarthritis or in the peri-articular tissues in inflammatory joint disease. Patients with fibromyalgia often have tender pressure points over soft tissues not related to any joint structures. Swelling of the joint is either within or around the joint and can either be a soft tissue, e.g. synovial swelling or effusion, or harder lesions such as osteophytes or rheumatoid nodules. Palpation of the joint during movement can demonstrate the presence of crepitus (course, rough clicks or cracks. This is suggestive of underlying articular cartilage damage.

Examination of the joint

Examination of the function of individual joints or groups of joints can be subdivided into those the patient can undertake and those elicited by the physician.

Active movement is when the patient undertakes the movement, and can give a guide as to the extent of movement that the patient finds feasible.

Passive movement is when the examiner undertakes this process; it can establish the complete range of movement, which in the normal circumstance is larger than active movement.

Gait, arms, legs and spine Detailed examination of the regions of the musculo-skeletal system should include the gait, upper limb (arm), lower limb (leg) and spine (GALS), and is best performed by asking the patient to mimic movements undertaken by the examiner.

Gait The gait examination can take place during entry to the examination room. While a symmetrical gait is usually normal, an asymmetrical (antalgic) gait is indicative of pathology on the affected side because the patients spends as little time on a painful leg as possible. A shuffling gait can suggest Parkinson's disease as a cause of stiffness. The use of a stick or other walking aid should be held in the contra-lateral hand to support the affected side.

Upper limb Examination of the upper limbs reflects their role, which is to place the hand in the correct position so that it can undertake its intricate functions (mouth for feeding, perineum for ablution) (see Table 3.2). Detailed examination of individual finger joints is usually not worthwhile but can show a specific site of pain such as the carpo-metacarpal joint of the thumb in

Table 3.2   Useful rapid examination for upper limbs

- Shoulder problems: Difficulty raising arms from resting position to the ears through abduction

- Elbow problems: Difficulty straightening elbows when held out in front of patient

- Wrist dysfunction: Difficulty holding hands in prayer position with elbows apart—finger flexion or wrist extension

- Poor hand function: Difficulty holding hands in prayer position
                          Inability to make a tight fist
                          Impaired ability to oppose thumb and little finger

osteoarthritis. Examination may reveal muscle wasting, the distribution of joint deformity and any skin or subcutaneous lesions. Examination of the metacarpophalangeal joints as a set may illicit pain and disability. Limitation of the power grip (failure to make a complete fist) or impaired precision grip (failure to oppose the thumb and little finger) are features of destructive inflammatory joint disease, such as rheumatoid arthritis. The association of distal interphalangeal joint disease with synovitis and limitation of function suggests a psoriatic arthropathy (Figure 3.2), whilst bony nodules (osteophytes) at this site (Figure 3.3) and minimal effect on function suggests nodular osteoarthritis.

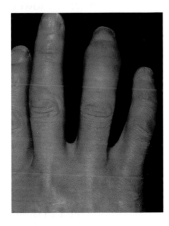

Figure 3.2 *Psoriatic arthritis hands*

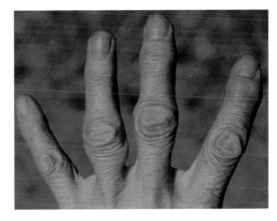

Figure 3.3 *Osteoarthritis nodules*

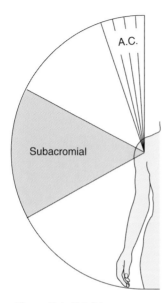

Figure 3.4 *Painful arc*

Asking the patient to raise their hands behind their neck or place them behind their back assesses the range of movement at the shoulder and elbow. Location of the exact site of pain and demonstration of limitation of specific movements (flexion/extension at the humero-ulnar joint) and rotation (at the upper radio-ulnar joint) can then be elicited if required. Of the range of movements at the shoulder flexion, extension, abduction and adduction are best examined with a straight arm while for internal and external rotation, the arm flexed at the elbow is used to show limitations. Examination of the face will demonstrate the presence of pain, such as that in the painful arc where flexing the shoulder to the upright position produces pain at the top of the arc in acromio-clavicular (A.C.) disease (Figure 3.4). Pain on progressive adduction of the arm to the torso between 80-120°, indicates a painful arc and is suggestive of supraspinatus tendinitis.

Lower limb Examination of the lower limb assesses the ability of the patient to transfer from one place to another by getting up from the lying or sitting position and walking (see Table 3.3). With the patient lying flat on the couch, examine for foot deformities in skin and bone. The foot is one of the commonest sources of poor lower limb function. The ankle is a regular site for damage because of ligament instability over the lateral malleolus following inversion injury. Assessment of active movement of the knee to 90° (both sides for comparison) also allows review for the presence of crepitus that can commonly be found between the patella and the underlying femur. Ligament instability can result from severe trauma and can be detected by passive movement against the force of the ligament: the lateral collateral ligament function is tested by forced adduction of the knee joint. Active knee flexion is only possible in the presence of a normal hip because it requires hip flexion to 45°, but internal rotation is often the first to be restricted in hip disease. Marked dysfunction of the hip joint leads to a positive Trendelenberg test where muscle weakness on the affected side resulting from long-standing disease causes the pelvis to tip downwards instead of rising on weight-bearing.

Table 3.3 Useful rapid examination for gait and lower limbs

General problems	Walk ten feet away from and towards the doctor
Hip problems	Positive Trendelenberg's sign Limited internal/external rotation Limited abduction and adduction
Knee problems	Muscle wasting Effusion filling in of peripatellar contours Patella tap Baker's cyst in popliteal area
Ankle problems	Examine arches while standing
Foot problems	Examine for callosities Deformities in MTP joints and toes

Spine The spine is best examined initially as a whole in the standing position looking for scoliosis or other deformity (see Table 3.4). More detailed examination should be undertaken in regions (cervical and lumbar), with the patient facing a mirror to allow the examiner to watch the facial expression. Palpation of the vertebral bodies can elicit local pain over a crushed vertebra and flexion and extension of the lumbar spine also allows examination of movements of the thoracic spine. Adequate intervertebral movement should be observed to exclude ankylosis. Limitation of lateral flexion and rotation

Table 3.4 Useful rapid examination for spine

• General examination	Examine for normal lordosis and also scoliosis Bend forwards and backwards Palpate for tender areas Look for muscle spasm
• Cervical spine	Flex sideways and look over both shoulders
• When lying supine	Limited straight leg raising—lower disc prolapse
• When lying prone	Limited leg extension (prone)—upper disc prolapse

can also be shown in lumbar and cervical spine in degenerative disease. The sacroiliac joints have only limited movement because of their partial fibrous nature. However, they may be palpated in the upright position, or when lying on the side, pressure of the pelvic rim can elicit tenderness over the sacroiliac region.

EXAMINATION OF SPECIFIC AREAS

Peri-articular tissues

Peri-articular tissues are common sites of pain but usually do not indicate significant inflammation within a joint. Location of bursae over various bony prominences such as the olecranon, greater tronchanter, patella and pre-patella ligament can be the site of bursitis. Pain at the tendon insertion (enthesitis) can play a part in local damage such as tennis or golfer's elbow (Figure 3.5), but are also seen particularly in psoriatic arthritis and other inflammatory joint diseases. Moving the limb against resistance will usually exacerbate the pain in these sites.

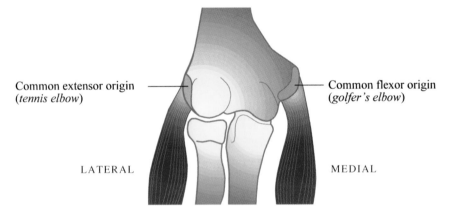

Common extensor origin (*tennis elbow*)

Common flexor origin (*golfer's elbow*)

LATERAL

MEDIAL

Figure 3.5 *Sites of pain in the elbow entheses*

Tenosynovitis

Tenosynovitis or inflammation of the tendon sheath can occur as a result of local soft tissue injury or as part of a systemic disease such as rheumatoid arthritis. Palpable tenderness often with fine crepitus over the lesion is characteristic of these lesions, such as in De Quervain's tenosynovitis (Figure 3.6) or in trigger finger.

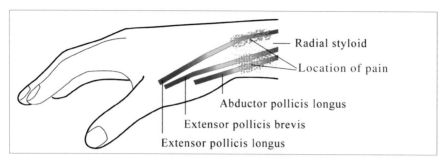

Figure 3.6 *De Quervain's tenosynovitis.*

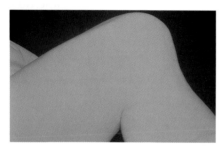

Figure 3.7 *Draw test for anterior cruciate ligament*

Ligament instability

Ligament instability is usually associated with tenderness over the insertion (enthesis) together with disruption of function of that ligament. For example in the knee joint, the medial and lateral collateral ligaments limit medial and lateral flexion of the straightened knee. Excessive strain on the medial ligament such as following a running or skiing injury can lead to ligament damage either at the enthesis or within the ligament structure itself. Forced lateral flexion at the knee will demonstrate laxity of movement and induce pain at the enthesis.

The anterior and posterior cruciate ligaments maintain anterior/posterior integrity of the knee during flexion. Rupture of the anterior cruciate ligament leads to posterior dislocation of the tibia so that the femur overrides the tibia at 90^{0} flexion (Figure 3.7). Loss of posterior cruciate ligament function leads to anterior dislocation of the tibia but only when the tibia is pulled forwards by pressure exerted from behind the knee. Local damage to ligaments holding the meniscal cartilage in place, produce pain and tenderness over the joint line, such as that seen in meniscal tears.

Complete system examination

Complete system examination of the patient may be necessary to exclude other diseases. Diseases of the neuromuscular system can produce pain and weakness from entrapment neuropathies or following neural ischaemia

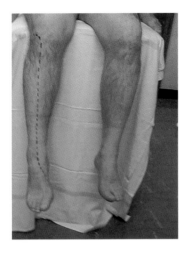

following vasculitis of the vasa nervorum (Figure 3.8). Equally, muscular dystrophy and myositis can also produce these symptoms. However, inflammatory joint disease can occur with lung fibrosis, inflammatory bowel disease, skin disease, and as a manifestation of renal disease that might be demonstrated during clinical examination.

Figure 3.8 *Foot drop in a patient with lateral popliteal nerve damage*

chapter 4

Investigation of the rheumatic diseases

The diagnosis in patients with symptoms of the rheumatic diseases is established by detailed history and careful examination (Table 4.1). Laboratory tests are helpful in confirming the clinical diagnosis but should not be used as a substitute for adequate history and examination, because few of these tests are specific.

Table 4.1 Useful screening investigations in rheumatic diseases

(To be interpreted with the clinical features)

- Haematology — Haemoglobin, white cell count
  ESR, ferritin

- Biochemistry — C-reactive protein (CRP)
  Renal and liver function tests
  Uric acid
  Calcium and phosphate
  Creatine phosphokinase (aldolase)
  Thyroid function tests

- Immunology — Rheumatoid factor
  Anti-nuclear antibody

- Radiology — x-ray of the affected joint

- Nuclear medicine — Bone scan imaging

COMMON SIMPLE INVESTIGATIONS

During active inflammation C-reactive protein (CRP) synthesis rises while that of albumin and fibrinogen fall. These changes are secondary to increased IL-6 synthesis during inflammation, resulting in an increase in plasma viscosity and an elevated erythrocyte sedimentation rate (ESR). Successful treatment of rheumatoid arthritis leads to a fall in CRP and ESR so they are useful for monitoring. In SLE there is often a rise in ESR that is out of proportion when compared to the CRP. In some patients with seronegative arthritides they may both be normal, but in general a normal CRP and ESR virtually excludes active systemic inflammation.

Haematology investigation

Haematology investigation of patients with chronic inflammatory diseases often shows a normochromic, normocytic anaemia. Blood loss from the gastrointestinal tract can lead to iron deficiency and malabsorption of vitamin B12 and folate can occur as a result of other autoimmune diseases producing a megaloblastic anaemia. A deficiency of all can indicate a poor diet because of severe hand deformity. Elevation of the white cell count occurs in septic arthritis, acute arthritides, systemic juvenile arthritis, vasculitides and patients receiving corticosteroid therapy. Leucopenia and thrombocytopenia occur in Felty's syndrome and SLE, but indicate possible bone marrow suppression in patients receiving disease modifying or immunosuppressive anti-rheumatic drugs.

Biochemical tests

Elevation of uric acid occurs in 10% of normal men, but indicates gout in association with appropriate symptoms. Renal function tests can deteriorate in patients with scleroderma, SLE or vasculitis because of renal damage as part of the disease process, but can indicate toxicity from non-steroidal anti-inflammatory agents or DMARD therapy for rheumatoid arthritis, particulary gold, penicillamine or cyclosporin. Abnormal liver function tests can indicate autoimmune liver disease, active rheumatoid arthritis, or toxicity from NSAIDs but can result from sulfasalazine, methotrexate and azathioprine toxicity. Creatine phosphokinase is raised in myositis, and is used to monitor severity in response to treatment. Hormonal investigations may be abnormal, as often more than one autoimmune disease can occur together. Thyroid function tests are particularly useful in excluding myxoedema as a cause of arthralgias and myalgias.

Serological investigations

Serum rheumatoid factors are present in 75% of cases of rheumatoid arthritis. However, they can be detected in 100% of synovial fluids examined. Rheumatoid factors are by no means specific for rheumatoid arthritis being present in a variety of infections and in autoimmune connective tissue diseases. However, when present with clinical features of rheumatoid arthritis they confirm the diagnosis. High titres are indicative of a poorer prognosis in rheumatoid arthritis.

Antinuclear antibodies

Antinuclear antibodies (ANA) are found in many connective tissue diseases with more than 95% of SLE patients having a positive ANA, but they are positive in autoimmune and malignant diseases as well as during some acute and chronic infectious so care is necessary in their interpretation. Low titre ANA are often found in the ageing population, and in this situation are less likely to have clinical significance.

The appearance of the ANA gives a guide to the antibody specificity and can assist with diagnosis. A homogeneous ANA is suggestive of antibodies against DNA (suggestive of SLE) or DNA binding proteins (histones) as in drug-induced SLE (Figure 4.1(a)).

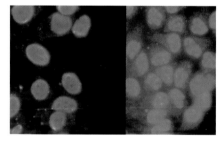

The speckled appearance (Figure 4.1(b)) suggests antibodies against the extractable nuclear antigens (RNA binding proteins) such as RNP and/or Sm (mixed connective tissue diseases or SLE) or Ro and/or La (Sjogren's syndrome and SLE). Other antibodies against the nucleolus are found in scleroderma and against the centromere are associated with limited systemic sclerosis (CREST).

Figure 4.1(a) *ANA homogeneous* and
Figure 4.1(b) *ANA speckled*

Anti-phospholipid antibodies

Anti-phospholipid antibodies are directed against cardiolipin, often in association with a protein antigen β^2-glycoprotein-1. Anti-cardiolipin antibodies were first detected in SLE, but are found in many autoimmune diseases and acute infections. They are significant in association with clinical features of the 'anti-phospholipid syndrome' (arterial or venous thrombosis, thrombocytopenia, recurrent fetal loss early in pregnancy). Anti-phospholipid antibodies inhibit *in vitro* blood coagulation assays, hence the term lupus anticoagulant, which is associated with a prolonged activated partial thromboplastin time that cannot be corrected by using a normal serum.

Rarely anticardiolipin antibodies can be associated with a more systemic illness, the so called catastrophic antiphospholipid syndrome with multiple organ infarction, acute respiratory distress, pulmonary hypertension and central nervous system failure.

Anti-neutrophil cytoplasmic antibodies

Anti-neutrophil cytoplasmic antibodies (ANCA) are detected using neutrophils as the target. If the antibody staining is cytoplasmic, it is known as c-ANCA, an antigen now identified as proteinase-3. These antibodies are found in about 80% of Wegener's granulomatosis patients and a few with microscopic polyarteritis.

Some ANCA stain a cytoplasmic antigen in a peri-nuclear pattern (p-ANCA). This is found in 40–50% of patients with microscopic polyarteritis and in other vasculitides but p-ANCAs are not specific being reported in other autoimmune diseases, during infections and in normal individuals.

Complement

Complement measurement is not routine but is useful in diagnosis and management of SLE. Low levels of C4 are common in the SLE population, probably because of a common partial genetic defect in the complement genes. However, persistently lower levels of C3 and C4 indicate activation of the classical complement pathway and in conjunction with the clinical condition can be helpful in monitoring disease activity in SLE.

Synovial fluid

Synovial fluid removal is useful to reduce symptoms when the joint is swollen, but synovial fluid analysis can be undertaken for diagnostic reasons. The presence of bacteria indicates septic arthritis, uric acid crystals (Figure 4.2) occur in gout and pyrophosphate crystals in pseudogout, Rheumatoid factor may be present in patients with seronegative rheumatoid arthritis.

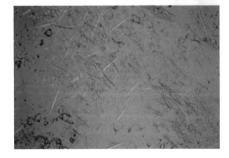

Figure 4.2 *Uric acid crystals*

Blood contamination can follow a traumatic tap but underlying diagnosis of villonodular synovitis, acute pyrophosphate arthropathy, haemophilia and Charcot's joints can lead to haemorrhagic taps.

Imaging of the joint

Imaging of the joint using standard radiography is useful in progression of osteoarthritis (bone sclerosis, loss of joint space, marginal osteophytes and bone cyst formation). Lateral views of the lumbar spine can also demonstrate degenerative changes, and confirm vertebral compression fractures and diseases of the intervertebral discs. Pelvis radiographs can detect sacroileitis (Figure 4.3).

X-rays in rheumatoid arthritis and other inflammatory joint diseases can demonstrate peri-articular osteoporosis, but subchondral erosions and reduced joint space indicates loss of cartilage in MCP and MTP joints and are diagnostic of rheumatoid arthritis. Subluxation and ankylosis occur in more chronic phases.

Ultrasound is increasingly used to image soft tissue, delineating ganglia (Figure 4.4) tenosynovitis, ligament rupture and bursitis with relative ease. However, even ultrasound appears normal in patients with fibromyalgia.

Computerised tomography (CT) is useful for disc prolapse but magnetic resonance imaging (MRI) is better and is increasingly used to evaluate soft tissue injuries around the shoulder and avascular necrosis of the hip, as well as meniscal tears and osteomyelitis. It is particularly helpful in evaluation of cervical spine disease in rheumatoid arthritis patients (Figure 4.5).

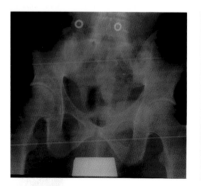

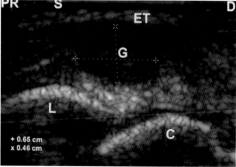

Figure 4.3 *Sacroileitis on pelvis*

Figure 4.4 *Ganglion* (G) *seen by ultrasound under extensor tendons* (ET) *above lunate* (L) *and cuneiform* (C)

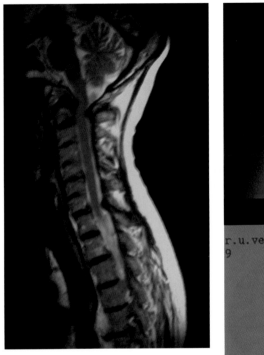

Figure 4.5 *Cervical spine disease in rheumatoid arthritis*

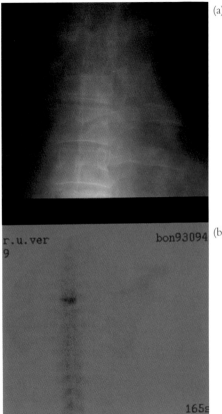

Figure 4.6 (a) *X-ray and* (b) *Bone scan on same patient showing vertebral collapse*

Radionucleotide scanning

Scintigraphy with technetium labelled bisphosphonate detects increased bone turnover by incorporation of radiolabelled bisphosphonate in new bone through osteoblastic activity. As such it is not diagnostic but can pick up metastatic deposits, osteoporotic vertebral collapse (Figure 4.6), diseases of bone (Paget's disease) and osteomyelitis as well as fractures that are difficult to visualise on x-ray. In addition, the increased peri-articular uptake is observed in inflammatory and degenerative arthropathies, however, the limited specificity requires abnormal bone scans should be correlated with x-rays. Radiolabelled white cell scans with gallium and indium can be used to localise infection and can be helpful in localising inflammatory bowel disease. Blood flow is being investigated using single proton emission computerised tomography (SPECT Scan) and may prove useful in patients with vasculitides and cerebral involvement with SLE.

Tissue biopsy

Tissue biopsy is undertaken to confirm clinical suspicion in a variety of connective tissue diseases. Muscle biopsy is important in establishing diagnosis of patients with primary muscle disease, such as muscular dystrophy or myositis (Figure 4.7). Synovial biopsy is diagnostic in the presence of infection (particularly TB) in the context of a monoarthropathy, and is a useful research tool for inflammatory arthropathy. Biopsy of the renal tissue can establish the degree and chronicity of glomerular and tubular tissue damage in patients with vasculitic or systemic lupus erythematosus. Finally biopsy of a clinically involved organ, such as skin, muscle, kidney, nerve or nasal mucosa, can be useful in establishing a diagnosis of vasculitis.

Figure 4.7 *Muscle biopsy in myositis (a) compared to normal muscle (b)*

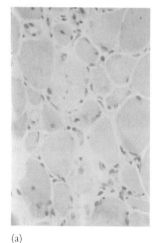

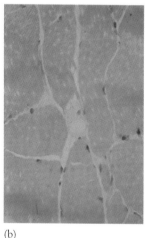

(a)   (b)

Part 2

COMMON AND IMPORTANT CONDITIONS

chapter 5

Osteoarthritis

Osteoarthritis is probably the single largest cause of physical disability and one of the commonest musculo-skeletal conditions seen in primary care. Despite its prevalence osteoarthritis has a very negative image with general practitioners and indeed with the general public.

There is a feeling that:

- osteoarthritis is inevitable with increasing age;
- there is no effective management;
- there is no point in going to the doctor: you just have to put up with it.

Increasingly these statements are being shown not to be true. Increasing age, while a risk factor, does not necessarily lead to the development of osteoarthritis, there are a number of effective management strategies for osteoarthritis, and increasing education of the primary care team should mean a much greater awareness of suitable interventions and much more support for individual patients.

The definition of osteoarthritis is often difficult and there is considerable controversy as to whether osteoarthritis can be diagnosed on clinical grounds alone or whether it requires x-ray confirmation. There is frequently poor correlation between x-ray changes and clinical symptoms and some patients may have gross x-ray changes with little in the way of symptoms while others may have considerable pain and stiffness with only minor radiological changes. From a practical point of view in primary care, clinical signs and symptoms are much more important than x-ray changes and an x-ray should only be requested if the result is going to change the management of the patient. It can sometimes be difficult to convince a patient, however, that an x-ray is not necessary and that careful examination of the affected joint will give much more useful information. As there are no investigations useful in osteoarthritis other than to exclude other conditions, it is sometimes tempting to x-ray the joint merely to be seen to be doing something although this is neither logical nor sensible.

PATHOPHYSIOLOGY

In the past osteoarthritis was thought of as a degenerative condition: a 'wear and tear' disease, which became worse with increasing age as joint surfaces inevitably broke drown. This view, however, has changed and osteoarthritis is now considered to be a dynamic condition, where breakdown of cartilage is followed by regeneration. The initial event is thought to be a localised breakdown of articular cartilage. At this area fibrillation develops due to changes in the proteoglycan matrix, with an increase in the water content and in the activity of the chondrocytes. Proteases and pro-inflammatory cytokines are thought to lead to tissue breakdown while at the same time causing inhibition of the tissue repair mechanisms. The impact-absorbing properties of this area decrease and the surface of the cartilage becomes roughened and irregular. There is then an increase in friction over this area resulting in thinning and eventual breaking down of the cartilage, possibly extending through to the bone. The joint then attempts repair by increasing blood supply and remodelling. At the margins of the joints, chondrocytes and osteophytes form, possibly to try to stabilise the joint and increase the articular surface. Changes also occur in the bone surrounding the joint, where sclerosis and bone cysts develop. Sclerosis occurs as new bone forms to strengthen the existing bony trabecular structure, and it is thought that these defects in the subchondral bone osteoblasts contribute to the onset and the progression of osteoarthritis. Bone cysts occur in areas where there is no articular cartilage and form as a result of raised intra-articular pressure, which is then transmitted into the marrow of the surrounding bone. These cysts may continue to enlarge until the pressure is equalised. These pathological changes of osteoarthritis are shown in Figure 5.1 with a normal joint for comparison.

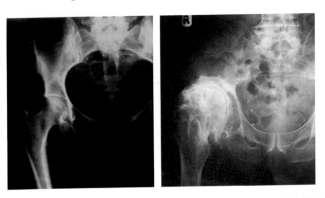

Figure 5.1 *Pelvis X ray showing* (a) *normal compared to osteoarthritic hip joints* (b)

Degradation products from cartilage, together with bone hydroxyapatite crystals, become deposited as debris in the joint space during the changes of regeneration. This debris may cause an inflammatory response, with the development of patchy areas of synovitis and increased viscosity of the synovial fluid. This inflammatory response may then cause ongoing destruction of joint tissue, leading in turn to effusion within the joint, raised intra-articular pressure, and eventual stretching and thickening of the joint capsule.

Synovial fluid does not merely provide lubrication in the joint, although this is one of its functions. It also appears to have a significant biological role and acts as a transport medium for nutrients and, along with the synovial membrane, may have hormonal and messenger functions. The main constituent of synovial fluid is a polymerised glycosaminaglycon or hyaluronan. In a normal joint, hyaluronan has a high molecular weight and this gives synovial fluid some of its biological properties of shock absorption and lubrication. It has also been suggested that the larger molecules in a normal joint exert some protective effect on the nociceptors or pain mediating receptors within joints.

In an osteoarthritic joint, synovial fluid has hyaluronan of smaller molecular weight. It is not yet clear whether this is the initial change which starts off the whole pathophysiological process of osteoarthritis or whether it is a secondary change occurring as the result of this process.

CLINICAL FEATURES

The clinical features of osteoarthritis reflect the pathological changes taking place within the joint. Pain is the main symptom of osteoarthritis. This typically occurs while using the joint or immediately after use, although in severe osteoarthritis pain may occur at rest and in particular in bed at night.

The pain of osteoarthritis is often difficult to describe and may be a deep dull ache or a sharp severe pain. A number of different pathological processes may give rise to the pain felt in an osteoarthritic joint as illustrated in Figure 5.2. These processes include:

- increased pressure within the capsule;
- increased pressure in the surrounding bone;
- inflammation of the synovial lining;
- peri-articular problems, such as bursitis or enthesopathies;
- alteration in muscle function around the joint;
- periosteal changes;
- abnormal pressure on the capsule and ligaments.

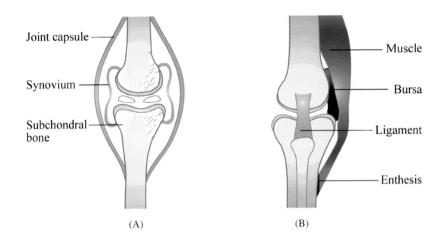

(A) (B)

Figure 5.2 *Sources of pain in osteoarthritis*

The pain of osteoarthritis is often accompanied by a degree of stiffness, which wears off fairly quickly as the joint is used, unlike the stiffness associated with inflammatory disease. Stiffness generally occurs after a spell of immobility, such as lying in bed or sitting, and is often described as 'gelling'. The pathological cause of the stiffness may be due to thickening of the capsule and alteration in the other peri-articular structures or to a degree of synovitis or effusion.

Joints affected by osteoarthritis often show a decrease in their range of movement probably due to bony changes and thickening of the capsule. Patients may also complain of a feeling that the joint is giving way due to weakness of the muscles surrounding the joint.

Coarse crepitus is a common feature in an osteoarthritic joint and is one of the clinical diagnostic features of osteoarthritis of the knee in the American College of Rheumatology Criteria (see Table 5.1). It can be felt on movement of the joint by both patient and examiner and is thought to be due to irregularities in the joint surface and osteophytes and chondrocytes at the joint edges preventing the normal smooth movement. Patients are often very concerned about crepitus but again this finding, though denoting pathological changes of osteoarthritis, is not necessarily associated with significant pain or disability.

Table 5.1 American College of Rheumatology classification criteria for osteoarthritis of the knee

Knee pain and radiographic osteophytes and at least one of the following three items:

- age over 50
- morning stiffness less than 30 mins in duration
- crepitus on motion

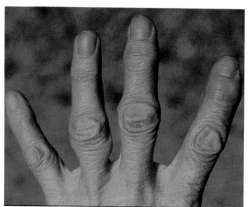

Figure 5.3 *Squaring of joint*

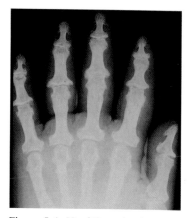

Figure 5.4 *Hand X ray showing Heberden's and Bouchard's nodes*

The growth of osteophytes at the joint margins causes bony swellings around the joint and clinically this leads to enlargement of the joint with changes in the appearance, often described as 'squaring' (Figure 5.3). When osteophytes are developing they can be tender and this is particularly evident in Heberden's nodes on the fingers (Figure 5.4)

Soft tissue swelling in an osteoarthritic joint may be due to a low–grade chronic synovitis and may be associated with an effusion. These are usually cool but may be warm during an inflammatory flare. Soft tissue swelling around the joint may also involve peri-articular structures, such as bursae.

In long-standing osteoarthritis, there may be eventual deformity of the joints due to destruction of the cartilage and changes in underlying bone and surrounding soft tissue. When this occurs in the medial compartment of the knee, it leads to a typical varus angulation or bowing. Inflammatory arthritis,

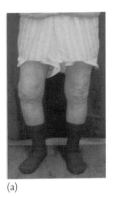
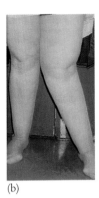

(a)   (b)

Figure 5.5 *Varus* (a) *and Valgus* (b) *angulation of the knee*

e.g. rheumatoid arthritis, on the other hand typically causes a valgus deformity (Figure 5.5)

Osteoarthritis is usually a slowly developing chronic disease although there may be spells of more rapid progression before the joint settles and becomes stable again. In some cases, however, progression can be rapid and patients can develop painful destructive changes over a relatively short space of time. This is sometimes seen in hip osteoarthritis, where patients can become severely disabled by pain and immobility over a short space of time. Joints can often show clinical, and occasionally radiographic, improvement. The outlook for many patients with osteoarthritis is good, and they are likely to suffer only intermittent problems of pain and reduced function. Often flares in symptoms can be related to over use of the joint due to some unaccustomed activity. Around half of all patients with osteoarthritis suffer daily joint pain and require a variety of interventions, while around 10% become increasingly incapacitated. The clinical features of osteoarthritis are shown in Table 5.2.

Table 5.2 Clinical features of osteoarthritis

• Pain on joint use	• Coarse crepitus
• Post-immobility stiffness	• Aged over 50
• Joint line tenderness	• Reduced range of movement of joint
• Bony swelling	• May be muscle-wasting

INVESTIGATIONS

There are no specific laboratory investigations for osteoarthritis. X-ray confirmation of the condition may be required, for example before surgical referral. Laboratory investigations and x-rays may be performed to exclude other conditions.

DIFFERENTIAL DIAGNOSIS

- Inflammatory arthritis,
- gout,
- other crystal arthropathy,
- mechanical problem within joint especially in knee, soft tissue problem around joint,
- fibromyalgia.

MANAGEMENT

Management of a patient with osteoarthritis should aim to:

- relieve pain;
- optimise function.

There are some lifestyle measures which have been shown to be effective in reducing pain and improving function. Education and information about the condition are essential in helping the patient to live with osteoarthritis and to manage their own condition. If the patient is overweight then weight loss is effective in reducing both pain and ongoing structural damage in knee osteoarthritis. Exercise is also very beneficial and patients should be told the difference between hurt and harm. Moving a joint within the limits of pain will not generally harm a joint affected by osteoarthritis and in most instances will in fact improve the condition. There are two main kinds of exercise: general aerobic exercise which improves general fitness, aids weight loss and often gives a feeling of wellbeing, and specific exercises which can improve the musculature round a specific joint e.g. quadriceps exercises for knee osteoarthritis. If the patient has osteoarthritis of the joints of the lower limb then wearing impact absorbing footwear can help to reduce the jarring through the leg when the heel strikes the ground. This can be achieved by wearing shoes such as trainers, which are flat with soft uppers, thick soft soles, and a wide forefoot. If trainers are not acceptable, then thin impact absorbing insoles available from sports shops may be used within the patient's normal footwear.

Most patients with osteoarthritis will require some form of pharmacological therapy at some stage of the disease. A suggested order for drug therapy in osteoarthritis is shown in Table 5.3.

Obviously patients will vary according to their response to particular drugs and their suitability for different therapies.

Other management options include:

- local heat or cold;

Table 5.3 Suggested order of drug therapy in osteoarthritis

- Paracetamol in adequate dose, i.e. 1gm qid
- Rubs, embrocations, topical NSAIDs
- Topical capsaicin
- Compound analgesics
- Oral anti-inflammatories—classical NSAIDs, COX 2 selective NSAIDs and COX 2 specifics or coxibs
- Other analgesics, e.g. tramadol, meptazinol
- Intra-articular steroid injection especially during an inflammatory flare
- Intra-articular hyaluronan injection for osteoarthritis knee

- rubs including NSAIDs bought from the pharmacy;
- physiotherapy including patellar taping, TENS, education and exercise therapy;
- occupational therapy for provision of aids and appliances and splints if appropriate;
- complementary therapy including homeopathy and acupuncture;
- glucosamine and chondroitin sulphate are amino monosaccharides that occur naturally within articular cartilage. They may have a long-term disease modifying effect, seem to be safe and appear to help osteoarthritic pain in some patients. They are not available on prescription in the United Kingdom but may be bought from health food shops. Chondroitin has a bovine origin, however, and this may be a cause for concern.
- Joint replacement – in severe OA, where the condition has a significant impact on a patient's life, joint replacement can provide major benefits in terms of pain relief and improved mobility.

REFERRAL

Most patients with mild to moderate OA will be managed within primary care provided there is access to physiotherapy and occupational therapy. Consider referral in the following circumstances:

- Doubt about the diagnosis.
- Specialized technique is required, e.g. some forms of steroid injection.
- Pain which is difficult to control.
- Consideration for surgery.

chapter 6

Rheumatoid arthritis

CLINICAL FEATURES

Rheumatoid arthritis is a symmetrical peripheral polyarthritis classically involving metacarpophalangeal and proximal interphalangeal joints (Figure 6.1), but equally affecting metatarsophalangeal joints in the feet. Specific criteria for the diagnosis of rheumatoid arthritis have been defined by the American Rheumatology Association (Table 6.1). However any synovial joint can be involved, including wrists, elbows, shoulders, ankles, knees, hips, cervical spine and temporo-mandibular joints (Figure 6.2). Symptoms include stiffness occurring early in the morning, improving as the day progresses, and pain is often described as toothache-like. Early in disease process the joint swelling is predominantly soft tissue with synovitis and/ or effusion, with heat because of joint inflammation. Deformity usually develops over years with joint destruction in the hands leading to ulnar deviation, volar subluxation of the metacarpophalangeal joints,

Table 6.1 American Rheumatology Association criteria for diagnosis of rheumatoid arthritis

RA is diagnosed when four or more of the following criteria are met.

- Morning stiffness of more than 1 hour for over six weeks
- Arthritis of three or more joint areas for six weeks
- Arthritis of the hand joints with swelling for over six weeks
- Symmetrical arthritis for six weeks or more
- Rheumatoid nodules
- Positive serum rheumatoid factor
- Characteristic radiographic changes of erosions

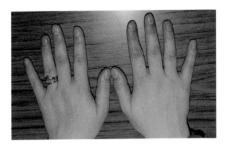

Figure 6.1 *Early rheumatoid arthritis hands*

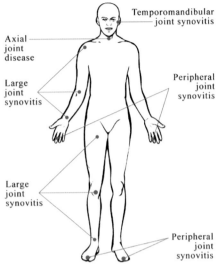

Figure 6.2 *Clinical pattern of rheumatoid arthritis*

Boutonniere's and Swan neck deformities in the fingers, Z-shaped thumb (Figure 6.3), fibular deviation of the toes. In the larger joints, fixed flexion deformities develop together with varus or valgus deformities dependent on the sites and degrees of joint destruction.

PRESENTATION

The clinical pattern of rheumatoid arthritis presentation and progression is variable. The onset can be explosive polyarthralgia that may last one to two years but can be followed by complete recovery. The insidious onset of palindromic rheumatoid arthritis is characterised by repeated brief attacks of synovitis and a positive circulating rheumatoid factor usually affecting one or more

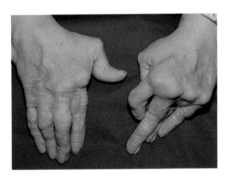

Figure 6.3 *Late rheumatoid arthritis (hands)*

joints, resolving rapidly. Other patients develop distinct episodes of relapsing and remitting disease with each acute episode being associated with further joint damage and progressive deformity. Severe chronic unresponsive disease, characterised by chronic deterioration of symptoms, which can result in the patient becoming wheelchair bound within five to ten years, is limited to around 5% of cases. The development of extra-articular disease features can occur at any time, but is more common in males, patients with positive rheumatoid factor and a genetic predisposition at the major histocompata-bility complex (MHC) (see below). At the present time none of these features can be differentiated at the beginning of the disease process, although those patients with a high ESR, circulating rheumatoid factor, and the shared genetic epitope, tend to be more severely affected.

JOINT PATHOLOGY

Synovial tissue is infiltrated with chronic inflammatory cells (Figure 6.4) which can be characterised as including activated T-cell lympho-cytes, B lymphocytes and mononu-clear cells of the monocyte/ macrophage lineage indicative of an ongoing local immune reaction. In addition local fibroblasts are also activated and most show evidence of new blood cell formation with activated endothelial cells. Inflam-matory and resident cells express

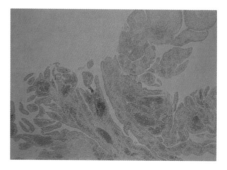

Figure 6.4 *Synovial histology*

general activation markers such as MHC class II, as well as their own identi-fying unique cell surface markers. Activated synovial macrophages produce pro-inflammatory cytokines (tumour necrosis factor (TNF), Interleukin-1 (IL-1) and Interleukin 6 (IL-6)). These cytokines stimulate prostaglandin production leading to local inflammation and metalloproteinases that destroy cartilage and bone. There is increasing evidence that interaction between the T cells, macrophages and resident cells can lead to over-production of cytokines such as IL-12, IL-15 and IL-18 which are important in the innate immune response.

The site at which the inflamed synovium covers the joint cartilage is known as the cartilage/pannus junction. The local destruction is thought to lead to cartilage damage and failure of adequate repair leads initially to erosions that can be seen developing on x-ray (Figure 6.5) eventually to complete cartilage loss and progressive erosion of bone. The eventual destruction of bone tissue results in uncorrectable joint deformity and failure of function (Figure 6.6). At the cartilage/pannus junction, macrophages and synoviocytes can be found secreting pro-inflammatory cytokines and metal-loproteinases, and chondrocytes are missing from their lacunae (Figure 6.7). Synovial fluid, by comparison, usually contains 300-2,000 x 10^6 white

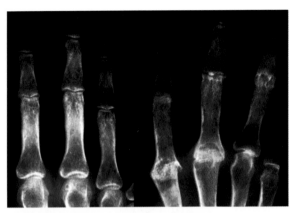

Figure 6.5 *X-ray of developing erosions*

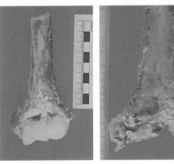

Figure 6.6 *Gross pathology of rheumatoid arthritis*

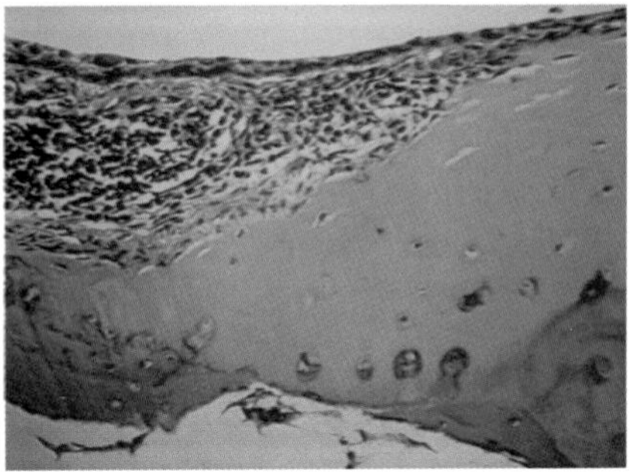

Figure 6.7 *Cartilage/pannus junction histology*

cells/L, predominantly neutrophils but activated lymphocytes and monocyte serious cells are found. Immune complexes containing rheumatoid factor are found in synovial fluid (SF) and can initiate cytokine production from macrophages.

LOCAL COMPLICATIONS OF SYNOVIAL JOINT DISEASE

Synovial hypertrophy leads to capsule and ligament stretching, hence exacerbating local deformity with ulnar deviation at the metacarpophalangeal joints (Figure 6.3), Boutonniere deformity (Figure 6.8), and swan neck deformities (Figure 6.9). However this can also press on local structures such as median nerve in the carpal tunnel, ulnar nerve at the medial epicondyle. Popliteal cysts (Baker cysts) may form in the posterior aspect of the knee joint. These can rupture, releasing inflammatory synovial fluid into the local tissue, which

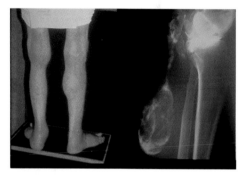

Figure 6.8 *Boutonniere deformity*

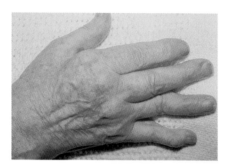

Figure 6.9 *Swan neck deformity*

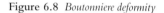

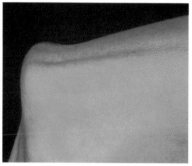

Figure 6.10 *Baker's cyst, right knee*

Figure 6.11 *Muscle wasting, left shoulder*

track into the calf, mimicking deep vein thrombosis (Figure 6.10). Synovial erosion through tendons can lead to rupture often affecting the long extensor tendons of the fingers. Severe joint involvement with rheumatoid arthritis can lead to joint fusion and subsequent muscle wasting (Figure 6.11).

EXTRA-ARTICULAR MANIFESTATIONS

Most extra-articular features of rheumatoid arthritis are rare and are demonstrated in Figure 6.12. When these features are present they can have implications on morbidity and indeed mortality of disease. When present they can be divided by specific system.

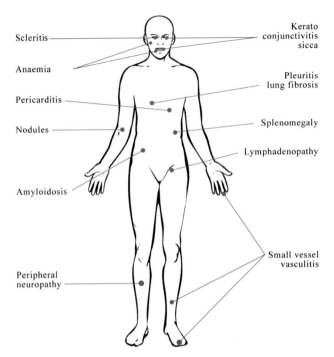

Scleritis

Anaemia

Pericarditis

Nodules

Amyloidosis

Peripheral neuropathy

Kerato conjunctivitis sicca

Pleuritis lung fibrosis

Splenomegaly

Lymphadenopathy

Small vessel vasculitis

Figure 6.12 *Pattern of extra-articular manifestations*

DERMATOLOGICAL MANIFESTATIONS

Rheumatoid nodules can be found in up to 40% of patients, often localised at sites of friction and extensor surface of the forearm, but can be found at the sacrum and subcutaneously over the Achilles tendon. Rheumatoid nodules (Figure 6.13) are associated with more severe disease and patients with

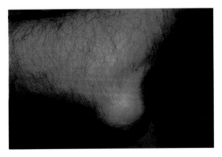

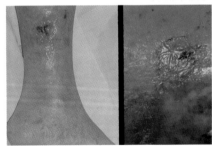

Figure 6.13 *Rheumatoid nodule*

Figure 6.14 *Leg ulcer (pyoderma gangrenosum)*

nodules are virtually always sero-positive for rheumatoid factor. Rheumatoid nodules commonly develop in patients receiving methotrexate therapy. Rheumatoid vasculitis is a vascular infiltration of lymphocytes with damage to small blood vessels. It can present with infarction resembling periungual splinter haemorrhages (Figure 6.1). Leg ulcers are usually localised to the lower half of the shins and can be venous, arterial or vasculitic in the aetiology. They can be a recurrent source of pain, disfigurement and infection. Pyoderma gangrenosum is a rare complication that can also cause leg ulceration (Figure 6.14).

OCULAR MANIFESTATIONS

Painful eyes in rheumatoid arthritis are usually due to secondary Sjogren's syndrome. After ten years the majority of patients have secondary Sjogren's syndrome with characteristic features of kerato-conjunctivitis sicca and necessitating local treatment. Scleritis (Figure 6.15) is a more sinister manifestation which can lead to scleromalacia (Figure 6.16) which can perforate, and can be a cause of visual loss. Drug toxicity can induce visual impairment, hydroxychloroquine rarely leading to maculopathy and glucocorticoids inducing cataracts.

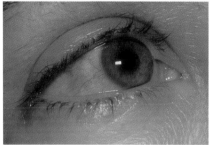
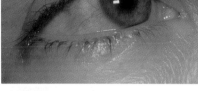
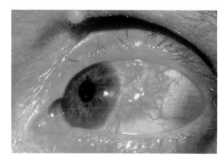

Figure 6.15 *Scleritis*   **Figure 6.16** *Scleromalacia*

NERVOUS SYSTEM

Peripheral neuropathy can result from local nerve compression, but rheumatoid vasculitis of small blood vessels can produce damage to the vasa nervorum producing a mononeuritis multiplex (Figure 6.17) and gold therapy can also produce a sensory peripheral neuropathy. Cervical spine involvement with synovitis at the atlanto-axial joint and facet joint articulations round the

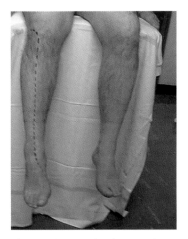

Figure 6.17 *Peripheral neuropathy –*
right lateral popliteal nerve damage

Figure 6.18 *MRI of cervical spine*
showing cord compression

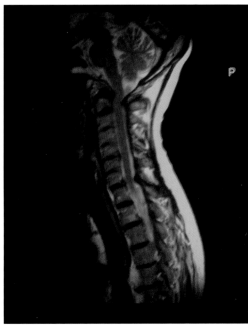

odontoid peg, can lead to atlanto-axial subluxation or superior subluxation of the odontoid peg through the foramen magnum, producing local compression on the upper cervical cord or brain stem (Figure 6.18). Joint destruction lower down the cervical spine can produce spondylolisthesis with compression of the cervical cord.

Respiratory involvement

Pleuritic chest pain can result from local pleural inflammation. Lung fibrosis can be seen on standard chest x-ray (Figure 6.19) and usually affects peripheral regions of the pulmonary architecture as seen on CT scan of the lung (Figure 6.20). Obliterative bronchiolitis can present with obstructive symptoms, but this is rare.

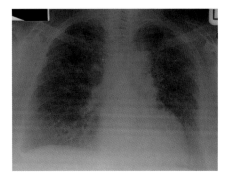

Figure 6.19 *Chest x-ray of lung fibrosis*

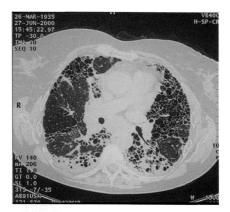

Figure 6.20 *CT scan of lung fibrosis*

CARDIAC INVOLVEMENT

Aseptic pericarditis occurs in about 33% of rheumatoid arthritis patients but is usually asymptomatic. Rheumatoid nodules can be found in cardiac tissue where, if it involves the conduction system, it can produce heart block.

HAEMATOLOGICAL MANIFESTATIONS

The commonest haematological feature is anaemia. While the normochromic normocytic anaemia associated with active phases of rheumatoid arthritis is common, chronic iron deficiency because of blood loss through the gastrointestinal tract is often a complication. There is an increased frequency of pernicious anaemia in rheumatoid arthritis patients because of the autoimmune nature of both diseases. Felty's syndrome is rare (around 1%), the accompanying splenomegaly neutropenia and rheumatoid arthritis is usually accompanied by severe synovitis and joint destruction, and often with the presence of other extra-articular features.

KIDNEY INVOLVEMENT

The kidney is rarely involved in rheumatoid arthritis unless there is secondary amyloidosis causing nephrotic syndrome. Gold and penicillamine can cause a membranous glomerulonephritis with proteinuria. Renal tubular acidosis is also a rare complication.

INVESTIGATIONS

Haematology

Full blood count, as anaemia and thrombocytosis are common during active phases of rheumatoid arthritis. White cell count and platelet count should be monitored during disease modifying drug therapy and immunosupressant therapy. The ESR correlates well with disease activity.

Biochemistry

Complement reactive protein (CRP) is usually increased and mimics disease activity. Alkaline phosphatase and gamma glutamyl transpeptidase (gamma GT) are often increased moderately during active phases of disease.

Immunology

IgM rheumatoid factor is positive in the serum in 75% of cases and is associated with more severe disease. The anti-nuclear antibody (ANA) is positive in up to 50% of patients.

Synovial fluid

Synovial fluid aspiration often shows elevated white cell count. Increased proteins and rheumatoid factor are found in virtually all cases of rheumatoid arthritis. Microbiological examination for bacteria should be carried out to exclude septic arthritis.

Diagnostic imaging

Joint radiography can demonstrate soft tissue swelling, joint space narrowing, peri-articular osteoporosis, bone erosions (Figure 6.5) as well as the underlying deformities. Cervical spine examination can demonstrate atlanto-axial subluxation. Chest x-ray can demonstrate pulmonary involvement (nodule and fibrosis). MRI is useful for imaging cervical spine in suspected cases of neurological involvement of the cervical cord (Figure 6.18). Diagnostic ultrasound is being increasingly used for examination of popliteal cysts, tendon rupture and other soft tissue damage.

EPIDEMIOLOGY

Rheumatoid arthritis affects 1–2% of the Caucasian population. Prior to the age of 50 rheumatoid arthritis is six times as common in females as in males. After the age of 50 this increase drops to 1.5:1. The prevalence increases with age, with the mean onset between 30 and 55. All races are involved but certain racial groups (Pima Indians) have a very high incidence of rheuma-toid arthritis. There is an increased incidence in urban black Africans compared to those living in rural communities.

AETIOLOGY

The cause of the autoreactive immune response in rheumatoid arthritis is unknown. Genetic susceptibility has been implicated by twin studies that show an increase in rheumatoid arthritis in monozygotic over dizygotic twins. This has been confirmed by the demonstration of an association with human leucocyte antigen DR4 and DR1. Rheumatoid arthritis is particu-larly common in DR4 subgroups DRβ 1*0401 and 0404 (Pima Indians have a high frequency of the DRβ 1*0404 allele) but family studies show that it is likely that genes other than those on chromosome 6 will also be involved. Although viral and bacterial causes have been implicated no conclusive evidence supports a role for Epstein Barr virus, parvovirus or e. coli in the aetiology of rheumatoid arthritis.

TREATMENT

In the absence of any cause for rheumatoid arthritis, treatment is empirically directed to alleviation of pain, suppression of active disease and conservation of joint function. A multidisciplinary team is central to effective treatment for patients with rheumatoid arthritis, to provide a dedicated programme of education and patient support at the social, financial and emotional level. This is centred in primary care as well as the hospital environment providing an integrated care programme.

GENERAL MANAGEMENT

This is designed to provide a balance between rest to alleviate symptoms and programmed rehabilitation to maintain joint mobility. Admission to hospital can be more beneficial than staying at home, partly by providing a more anodyne environment, but also by giving access to comprehensive rehabilita-tion services.

Adequate supervision is essential to prevent flexion contractures during bed rest, by judicious use of intra-articular corticosteroids (triamcinolone or depomedrone) and appropriate splints. Previously formed contractures can also be corrected in this way, but cannot improve if they have been present for too long. Repeated injections at short intervals should be avoided unless designed to alleviate symptoms immediately prior to joint replacement.

Adaptation of the home environment (provision of cooking aids, extra stair rails, raised seating and bathroom adaptation) can facilitate activities of daily living and enable the patient to be maintained within their home environment. Provision of financial assistance through social services can provide financial support for carers and patients alike.

MEDICAL MANAGEMENT
Non steroidal anti-inflammatory drugs (NSAID)

These decrease the synthesis of prostaglandins and prostacyclins by inhibiting the enzyme cyclo-oxygenase that is found in excess in inflamed synovial tissue. Hence they are particularly indicated for inflammatory joint disease. Common examples include indomethacin, naproxen, diclofenac, sulindac, etodolac, nabumetone and ibuprofen.

Side effects These vary between drugs. The commonest include dyspepsia, nausea, tinnitus, headache and deterioration of renal function. The more severe include intestinal bleeding, stomach ulceration, hypersensitivity reactions and blood dyscrasias. The gastrointestinal effects are secondary to inhibition of cyclo-oxygenase in the stomach mucosa where a protective effect is observed. Removal of this protection leads to increase in gastrointestinal ulceration.

Monitoring No specific monitoring is recommended for NSAID use, but a check on haemoglobin and renal function is not inappropriate.

COX-2 inhibitors

Most non-steroidal anti-inflammatory agents inhibit production of both protective prostaglandins in the stomach and damaging prostaglandins within the synovial tissue. The enzymes responsible for the synthesis of these molecules are called cyclo-oxygenase (COX). COX 1 is responsible for synthesis of the protective prostaglandins and COX 2 responsible for those produced within the synovial tissue. Recent drug company research has concentrated on producing targeted molecules which inhibit COX 2 molecules, hence preferentially reducing synovial tissue prostaglandin production whilst maintaining production within the gastrointestinal mucosa. New drugs such as rofecoxib and celecoxib have reduced instance of ulcer formation, however, the patients can still develop dyspepsia and renal problems whilst taking these new drugs.

Disease modified anti-rheumatic drugs (DMARDs)

These drugs suppress synovitis in rheumatoid arthritis. They do not act immediately, taking up to six months to produce an adequate response and are also known as slow acting anti-rheumatic drugs (SAARD). They also improve pain, stiffness and suppress the acute phase response and most have been shown to reduce the rate of erosive disease development on x-ray. Treatment is preferentially started at the beginning of disease to minimise joint destruction.

Gold therapy

Sodium aurothiomalate is given initially in weekly intra-muscular injections of 50mg until there is a clinical and serological improvement, or for 20 weeks, which ever is the shorter. A test dose of 10mg is used to ensure no allergic reaction prior to commencement of the course. The 50mg dose is then dropped to fortnightly, three weekly and eventually monthly. Some patients can be maintained on six-weekly doses. Oral gold therapy is less effective than intramuscular treatment, but can be used if there is a needle phobia.

Side effects These include mouth ulcers, skin reaction, proteinuria, blood dyscrasia. Oral gold treatment is associated with looser bowel motions.

Monitoring Urine and blood should be tested one week prior to the gold injection to exclude the presence of proteinuria, leucopenia, and thrombocytopenia.

Penicillamine

This is a derivative of penicillin, but is not contraindicated in those with penicillin allergy. The dose commences at 125mg/day, increasing in doses of 125mg monthly to a maximum of 1000mg, or until a response as been obtained.

Side effects These include hypersensitivity skin reactions, nausea, loss of taste, mouth ulcers, skin reactions, proteinuria and blood dyscrasias. Rarely penicillamine can induce features of other autoimmune diseases including myasthenia gravis and drug induced SLE.

Monitoring Full blood count and urine should be checked on a weekly basis at the beginning of therapy for proteinuria, leucopenia and thrombocytopenia. Once a stable dose has been reached this can be undertaken monthly.

Sulfasalazine

This is a 'designer drug' consisting of aminosalicylic acid and the antibiotic sulfapyridine. This is given in 500mg doses daily, increasing up to 3gm/day by increasing in 500mg increments on a weekly basis. The total dose should ideally not exceed 40mg/kg.

Side effects These include nausea, vomiting, headache, blood dyscrasia, urine discolouration.

Monitoring Initially full blood count and liver function tests should be undertaken weekly as the dose is increasing. Thereafter monthly for three months and subsequently four times per year.

Hydroxychloroquine

This antimalarial agent is well tolerated with minimal side effects. Hydroxychloroquine is started at 400mg/day until response has been obtained and then the dose is reduced to a minimal level, usually 200mg three times/week.

Side effects Headache and visual disturbances can occur. Blood dyscrasias are rare. The major concern has been irreversible retinal damage, but this is so rare that ophthalmologists do not now routinely recommend monitoring of hydroxychloroquine therapy.

Monitoring Ideally all patients should have a full ophthalmic examination before treatment to ensure there are no contraindications to therapy. If examination can be arranged on an annual basis then this reassures the patient and physician accordingly.

Methotrexate

This folic acid analogue is extremely effective in rheumatoid arthritis. Long term studies show that more patients remain on methotrexate longer than other drugs. Dose regimes vary. Most rheumatologists start at a small dose (10mg/week) building up in 2.5mg increments until a response has been obtained.

Side effects Methotrexate can produce nausea and mouth ulceration and rarely myeloid suppression or pneumonitis.

Monitoring Full blood count and liver function tests are undertaken weekly until a stable dose is maintained, thereafter on a monthly basis.

Drug interactions Avoid trimethoprim and septrin.

Immunosuppressants

These agents are commonly reserved for patients with severe extra-articular manifestations of rheumatoid arthritis, or for those where standard treatment has been tried and treatment regimes exhausted. It is not recommended that patients taking immunosuppressants should receive live vaccinations as these might lead to active infections.

Azathioprine

Azathioprine is a purine analogue given in a maximum dose of 2.5mg/kg. The dose is usually commenced at 25 or 50mg/day increasing to the maximum dependent on response.

Side effects Nausea, vomiting, mouth ulceration, myeloid suppression and hepatotoxicity are seen.

Monitoring Full blood counts are undertaken, initially weekly dropping to monthly once a stable dose has been reached.

Cyclosporin-A

This reagent was developed from a fungal protein and used to prevent transplant rejection. It inhibits signalling within activated lymphocytes. It is used in doses of 2.5–4mg/kg.

Side effects These include nausea, vomiting and hepatotoxicity. There can be a dose-related impairment of glomerular renal function.

Monitoring Full blood counts are undertaken initially weekly dropping to monthly once a stable dose has been reached. Renal function should not reduce by more than 30% and hypertension may occur and require treatment.

Leflunomide

This recent addition to the rheumatologists armamentarium interferes with lymphocyte DNA synthesis. It is given in a loading dose of 100mg/day for three days and subsequently 20mg/day. It is reported to have a more rapid therapeutic effect than standard DMARD therapy.

Side effects These include nausea, diarrhoea, alopecia, neutropaenia and abnormal liver function tests.

Monitoring Full blood counts and liver function tests are undertaken fortnightly, reducing to every four and eight weeks after three and six months. The dose is reduced if liver function tests rise by two to three-fold and is stopped if the increase is above three-fold.

Drug interactions   Avoid phenytoin, warfarin and hepatotoxic drugs.

Cyclophosphamide

This alkylating agent is usually given in hospital practice and is generally restricted to use for patients with severe extra-articular features of disease which have produced significant end organ damage. It can be given as intravenous boluses or in oral form as weekly boluses or daily. It must be given in association with mesna to reduce side effects.

Side effects   These include myeloid suppression, infertility and malignancy. There is an increased risk of bladder toxicity with cystitis that can be reduced by ensuring high urine output during administration, but if cystitis develops there is an increased risk of bladder malignancy. Animal experiments suggest that the use of mesna reduces production of the toxic metabolite responsible for bladder irritation, and reduces the risk of cystitis and further malignancy.

Monitoring   Weekly full blood count and assessment for haematuria should be undertaken.

Combination therapy

Recent studies have shown benefit from use of combinations of DMARDs. The first showed a benefit of low dose methotrexate, sulfasalazine and hydroxychloroquine, over the use of single agents, and claimed to have a reduced side effect profile because of the smaller doses involved. Other investigations have suggested the usefulness of cyclosporin-A and sulfasalazine in combination. Combination of DMARD with prednisolone is not an uncommon combination in regular use.

This area will be the subject of future study to confirm the benefits of combination treatment.

Corticosteroids

Despite their use for over 50 years, the role for glucocorticoids in treatment of rheumatoid arthritis remains controversial. They undoubtedly have a potent anti-inflammatory effect, but doses needed for adequate therapeutic effect are unacceptably high. Recent studies have shown that when used in combination with standard DMARD therapy there is reduction in joint erosion on x-ray, but that the subjective improvement in patient symptoms and health assessment is not maintained beyond two years. The dose used is usually below 10mg prednisolone/day, but even at this level the effects of gluconeogenesis and the weak mineralocorticoid effects can be manifest.

Side effects Protein breakdown leads to muscle and skin atrophy, and osteoporosis due to bone matrix destruction, and is associated with hyperlip-idaemia and the characteristic fat redistribution. Enhanced glucose synthesis leads to cataract formation, impaired glucose tolerance and diabetes, and the mineralocorticoid effects lead to fluid retention, glaucoma and hypertension, and may be involved in changes in mental function. Impaired immune function leads to susceptibility to infection and possible reactivation of *Mycobacterium Tuberculosis* (MTB), and prolonged use suppresses the hypothalamic pituitary axis.

Monitoring Measurement of blood pressure and checks on plasma glucose and lipid levels are undertaken. Measurements of bone mineral density show rapid reduction after commencement of prednisolone; appropriate prophy-laxis with bisphosphonates is recommended.

New anti-rheumatic agents

Novel agents are being developed as a result of recent research. These include genetically engineered antibodies that are targeted to destroy T cells that infiltrate into the inflamed synovium. Although initial studies showed these agents to be effective, toxicity has limited their use, but it is hoped that newer generations of these agents could be designed to have reduced side effects.

Other agents block the action of tumour necrosis factor or Interleukin-1. Anti-TNF therapy has a particularly profound rapid action, reducing synovitis and the acute phase response within days of administration. Dose regimes are presently being worked out, but some can be administered on a daily basis subcutaneously, others are given intravenously, and appear to have synergistic effect with other drugs such as methotrexate. There are, however, reports of increased risk of infection and concerns about lymphoid malig-nancy. Interleukin-1 receptor antagonist has less effect on the acute phase response but this and anti-TNF therapy both reduce the greater development of erosive disease.

Surgical reconstruction

Surgical interventions are dealt with in detail elsewhere, but should be included as part of the multidisciplinary integrated care package. Reasons for surgical intervention are summarised in Table 6.2. Synovectomy either open or through an arthroscope can assist with management of a single problem joint. Synovial decompresssion can assist with local entrapment of nerves and

Table 6.2 Reasons for joint surgery in rheumatoid arthritis

- Pain   • Loss of function   • Instability

tendons and tendon repair may be required if rupture occurs. Osteotomy can help with forefoot pain (Keller's or Fowler's operations), and excision arthroplasty can help improve elbow joint function after removal of the radial head. Fusion can assist with deformity and pain particularly in the wrist, and ankle joints. However, the commonest surgical procedure is large joint replacement for premature joint failure with beneficial effects on pain and joint movement. Indications for replacement include immobility, nocturnal pain, and severe deformity.

PROGNOSIS IN RHEUMATOID ARTHRITIS

The course is variable, within ten years over 50% of patients are out of work, and this figure rises with increasing social deprivation.

After ten years, only 5-10% are severely crippled, a figure rising to 20% at 20 years. A poor prognosis is linked with insidious disease onset, early development of extra-articular disease manifestations, high titre of rheumatoid factor, and over 12 months of active disease without remission (Table 6.3).

Life expectancy is reduced by up to 15 years with five-year survival reduced by 50% in patients with severe disease with extra-articular features. This places this subgroup of rheumatoid arthritis patients into the same prognostic group as patients with triple vessel coronary disease and stage IV Hodgkin's disease.

Table 6.3 Poor prognostic features in rheumatoid arthritis

• Young disease onset	• Low haemoglobin
• Systemic manifestations	• Subcutaneous nodules
• Persistently high acute phase response	• Positive rheumatoid factor
	• Early erosive changes

EPIDEMIOLOGY

Assuming an average size of 2,500 patients, each GP will have approximately 25 cases of rheumatoid arthritis in their practice.

REFERRAL IN RHEUMATOID ARTHRITIS

Patients should be referred for:
- assessment of acute synovitis;
- commencement of DMARD therapy;
- assessment of disease complications;
- assessment of drug complications;
- review of active phases of disease process.

chapter 7

Crystal arthritis

INTRODUCTION

Deposition of various types of crystals can lead to classical arthritis.

■ Gout is caused by deposition of uric acid crystals, usually affecting the big toe.
■ Pseudogout commonly affects the knee and results from calcium pyrophosphate dihydrate (CPPD) deposition.
■ Deposition of calcium phosphate (apatite) usually affects the knee and shoulder.
■ Rarer varieties include cholesterol, oxalate, xanthine, and cysteine.

GOUT

Clinical features

Acute gouty arthritis usually presents as a monoarthritis (Figure 7.1) classically affecting the big toe (in 50% of cases). Symptoms produce the classic signs of inflammation, erythema, swelling, redness, heat, pain and loss of movement (Figure 7.2). The attack often starts with severe pain usually at night but rarely lasts more than two weeks. Between acute attacks the patient is asymptomatic, but 60% of patients have a further attack in the first year.

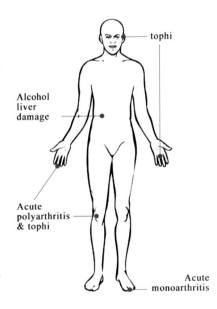

Figure 7.1 *Distribution of the clinical features of gout*

tophi

Alcohol liver damage

Acute polyarthritis & tophi

Acute monoarthritis

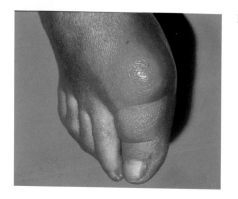

Figure 7.2 *Acute gout in big toe*

Causes of gout

Acute attacks result from uric acid crystal formation in synovial fluid (Figure 7.3) and also within synovial membrane and cartilage. Hyperuricaemia (above 420μmol/l in males and 360μmol/l in females) is the sole factor that predisposes to acute attacks of gout. Uric acid comes from purines derived from DNA breakdown and hyperuricaemia usually results from reduced uric acid

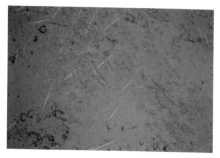

Figure 7.3 *Uric acid crystals under polarised light*

excretion. However, 10% of males have asymptomatic hyperuricaemia, but only 10% of these patients go on to develop gout.

Predisposing factors to gout include high social status, older age, obesity, diabetes mellitus, high alcohol consumption, lead poisoning, hypertension, ischaemic heart disease and type IV hyperlipidaemia (Table 7.1).

If gout is not treated, serum urate crystals will deposit outside the joint producing:

- uric acid stones: 10-25% of patients with gout, avoid dehydration or low urine pH (diarrhoea, ileostomy);
- interstitial renal damage results from a combination of tubular obstruction, infection, stone formation and glomerulosclerosis;
- tophi formation in subcutaneous tissues: cartilage of the ear (Figure 7.4), skin at sites of pressure and in tendons;
- tophi formation in synovial tisssues: leading to chronic arthritis (Figures 7.1, 7.5) with x-ray damage (Figure 7.6).

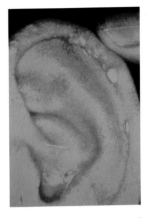 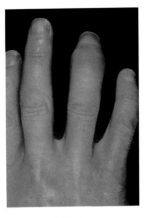 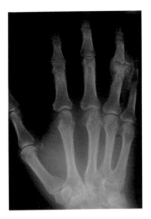

Figure 7.4 *Tophi on pinna of ear*   Figure 7.5 *Tophaceous gout*   Figure 7.6 *x-ray of tophaceous gout*

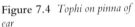

Table 7.1 Causes of raised uric acid

(males < 420µmol/l females <360µmol/l)

Primary   reduced clearance with normal kidney function
           over-production because of enzyme deficiency

Secondary reduced clearance
                   renal failure
                   lead poisoning
                   diuretic therapy
           inhibition of excretion
                   starvation
                   alcohol excess
                   acidosis (diabetic or lactic)
           overproduction
                   enzyme deficiencies
                   myelproliferative disorders
                   obesity
                   severe psoriasis

Investigations

Haematology Raised ESR, haemoglobin normal, white cell count normal or neutrophilia.

Biochemistry Uric acid is elevated in 90% of cases (it can be normal during acute attacks). Urea/creatinine level is raised in renal failure; auto-antibodies are negative.

X-ray This will only demonstrate erosive changes later, after recurrent attacks.

Synovial fluid haematology White cell count (neutrophils) is high ($>100,000 \times 10^6/l$).

Microbiology Gram stain and culture should be normal.

Microscopy Needle-shaped negatively birefringent crystals will be seen under polarised light (Figure 7.3).

Differential diagnosis

These include septic arthritis, peri-articular cellulitis, local bursitis and oligo-articular psoriatic arthritis.

Management of gout

40% of acute gout is characterised by only one attack. Indomethacin or suitable non-steroidal anti-inflammatory agents can be used, but if contraindicated then colchicine is helpful. Intra-articular injection of corticosteroids may be needed.

Only repeat acute attacks and the presence of tophi require prolonged treatment. Dietary advice can prove beneficial (Table 7.2), however, this is usually only of limited value. In all cases NSAIDs or colchicine should be used to suppress the acute attack, and continued alone for at least six weeks.

Table 7.2 Dietary advice for patients with gout and uric acid stones

- Lose weight
- Avoid purine rich foods (meats, fish)
- Avoid excess alcohol
- Avoid diuretics and aspirin
- Drink adequate fluids
- Eat more low purine foods (vegetables, cheese)

Table 7.3 Treatment of acute gout

- Dietary advice as in Table 7.2
- Any non-steroidal anti-inflammatory drug
- Colchicine 1mg stat. and 0.5mg 2-hourly until toxicity
- Corticosteroid injection if oral therapy not indicated
- Allopurinol 300-600mg/day (with NSAID cover)
- Probenecid
- Monitoring
- Maintain uric acid level below 420mmol/l

Allopurinol should then be added in combination with the NSAID for a further few weeks (to prevent acute attacks precipitated by allopurinol). The NSAID should then be tailed off leaving the patient on allopurinol alone (Table 7.3). The aim should be to maintain the serum uric acid level within the normal range by titration of the allopurinol dose. If treatment is successful, the tophi should disappear, albeit slowly.

Repeat attacks while apparently taking allopurinol usually occur because of failure to comply with therapy or following binge drinking. These should be managed with NSAID or colchicine therapy.

Uricosuric agents (probenecid or sulfinpyrazone) can assist with lowering the uric acid level but should be avoided in the presence of renal failure and urolithiasis.

Asymptomatic hyperuricaemia

As 10% of males have elevated serum uric acid, its presence does not guarantee acute attacks of gout. Allopurinol therapy is needed if there is a family history of renal stones or repeated uric acid levels over double normal range in clear-cut cases of uric acid over-production.

Epidemiology

Assuming a practice size of 2,500 patients, each GP will have 125 males with asymptomatic hyperuricaemia, but only 15 males and four females with gout. There is an increasing recognition of gout in elderly females because of the increased use of loop diuretics (Table 7.1).

PSEUDOGOUT
Clinical features

Calcium pyrophosphate dihydrate (CPPD) deposition is a common cause of acute monoarthritis in middle-aged and elderly females. Deposition of CPPD crystals within the menisci can be an asymptomatic finding in chondrocalcinosis, but may occur on top of osteoarthritis. The arthropathy usually affects the knees or wrists and is often precipitated by a second trigger such as trauma, surgery or illness (Figure 7.7). Between attacks the patients is usually asymptomatic, but sub-acute attacks can occur, affecting wrists, knees and elbows mimicking rheumatoid arthritis with early morning stiffness, pain and deformity.

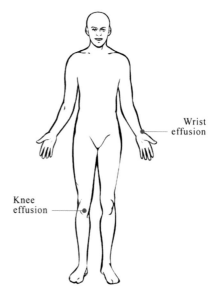

Figure 7.7 *Distribution of pseudogout*

Predisposing causes for pseudogout

There are familial causes of pyrophosphate deposition, but others include haemochromatosis, hypercalcaemia, hyperparathyroidism, hypothyroidism, ochronosis and Wilson's disease.

Investigations

Haematology Raised ESR, white cell count normal or neutrophilia .

Biochemistry Urea/creatinine level is raised in renal failure. Auto-antibodies are negative.

X-ray This will show chondrocalcinosis in menisci and triangular cartilage. Features of underlying osteoarthritis are also common (Figure 7.8).

Synovial fluid haematology White cell count (neutrophils) is high ($>100,000 \times 10^6/l$).

Microbiology Gram stain and culture are normal.

Microscopy Rectangular weakly positive birefringent crystals will be seen (Figure 7.9).

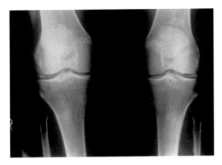

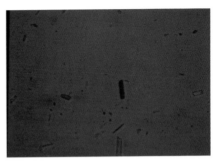

Figure 7.8 *X-ray of chondrocalcinosis*

Figure 7.9 *Pyrophosphate crystal under polarised light*

Management of acute arthritis

Management with joint aspiration, identification of pyrophosphate crystals (Figure 7.8), exclusion of septic arthritis, treatment with NSAIDs, colchicine or intra-articular steroids is appropriate. The lesion is usually self-limiting after two weeks. If clinical and x-ray evidence suggest severe osteoarthritis joint replacement should be considered.

CALCIUM PHOSPHATE CRYSTAL DEPOSITION (HYDROXYAPATITE)

Milwaukee shoulder/knee

This hydroxyapatite associated destructive arthropathy is usually seen in elderly females. The shoulders and knees are the main joints affected with sudden onset of pain and swelling, usually on the dominant side. There is a large cold effusion, variable pain on movement of the joint and rapid development of joint destruction and subluxation.

Investigations

X-ray This will show rotator cuff defects with upward migration and destruction of humeral head but little or no bone remodelling and no changes of osteoarthritis.

Synovial fluid haematology There is a low white cell count.

Microbiology Gram stain and culture is normal.

Microscopy Numerous CPPD and hydroxyapatite crystals will be seen.

Treatment

Analgesics, NSAIDs and physiotherapy are all beneficial to some degree. Regular joint aspiration and corticosteroids may be necessary, and surgical replacement may be needed.

OTHER CRYSTAL ASSOCIATED ARTHROPATHIES

Xanthine is a rare cause of acute arthritis with renal calculi.
Cholesterol crystals can be associated with chronic synovial effusions in rheumatoid arthritis and osteoarthritis (Figure 7.10).
Cysteine crystal formation can precipitate a crystal arthritis.

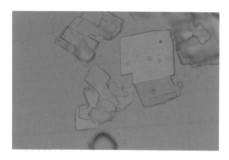

Figure 7.10 *Cholesterol crystal*

chapter 8

Seronegative spondarthritides

INTRODUCTION

The term seronegative spondarthritides covers a variety of different conditions with common articular, extra-articular and genetic features (Table 8.1), but as IgM rheumatoid factor is not a feature in these patients they are deemed seronegative. There is usually a strong family history and a common genetic background as many patients carry the HLA-B27 antigen. However, as this is present in approximately 9% of Caucasians in the United Kingdom and the incidence of the spondyloarthropathies is approximately 1%, other genetic factors must be involved. It is postulated that the arthropathy develops secondary to an underlying infection at a distant site such as the gut or genital tract.

Table 8.1 The spondyloarthritides

* Ankylosing spondylitis
* Enteropathic-acquired reactive arthritis
* Sexually acquired reactive arthritis
* Enteropathic arthritis

ANKYLOSING SPONDYLITIS

This is characterised by onset of back pain usually localised at the lower one-third of the back, with early morning stiffness sometimes radiating to the buttocks or thighs. There is often a strong family history not only of ankylosing spondylitis (Figure 8.1) but also a greater family incidence of psoriasis and inflammatory bowel disease. Early signs include limitation of

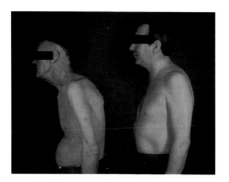

Figure 8.1 *Ankylosing spondylitis father and son*

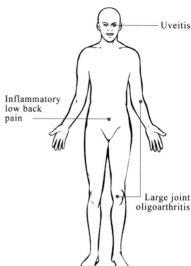

Uveitis

Inflammatory low back pain

Large joint oligoarthritis

Figure 8.2 *Clinical pattern of ankylosing spondylitis*

forward and lateral flexion, pain over the sacroiliac joints and on compression thereof and failure to obliterate the lumbar lordosis on forward flexion.

Extra spinal features include a lower limb mono- or oligo-arthritis that is seen in up to 40% of patients (Figure 8.2). Single lower limb large joint arthritis is not an uncommon method of presentation in boys aged 10-16. Uveitis (Figure 8.3) with photophobia, blurred vision and a painful red eye occurs in up to 25% of patients and is a medical emergency. Inflammation of tendon and ligament insertions (enthesitis) is common, and can often be detected at the site of the calcaneus (Figure 8.4) as is pain at the site of the costochondral junction. Amyloidosis, aortic regurgitation, cardiac conduction defects and apical pulmonary fibrosis are all rare extra-articular manifestations in ankylosing spondylitis (Table 8.2).

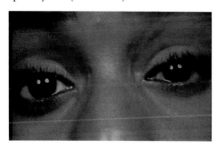

Figure 8.3 *Uveitis*

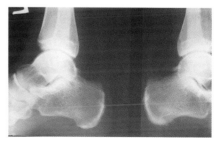

Figure 8.4 *X-ray of heel*

Table 8.2 Extra-articular features of ankylosing spondylitis

• Iritis / uveitis	• Cardiac conduction defects
• Aortic regurgitation	• Atlanto-axial subluxation
• Amyloidosis	• Cauda-equina syndrome
• Osteoporosis	• Apical pulmonary fibrosis

Investigations

Haematology Raised ESR, but haemoglobin, white cell count and ESR can be normal.

Biochemistry Raised CRP which mimics ESR.

Immunology Rheumatoid factor and ANA are universally negative. IgA may be raised. HLA-B27 is more common than in the normal population (around 95%)

X-ray Sacro-iliitis is commonly present at presentation (Figure 8.5). There may be ossification of anterior longitudinal ligament. Syndesmophyte formation leads to the typical bamboo spine (Figure 8.6). Erosive changes can be seen at the synthesis pubis.

There is a fluffy appearance at entheses and tuberosities of the pelvis (Figure 8.5).

Synovial fluid haematology White cell count is high ($>10,000 \times 10^6/l$).

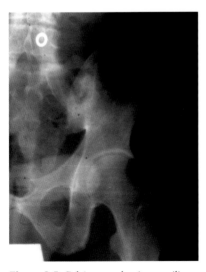

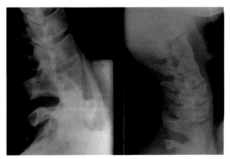

Figure 8.5 *Pelvis x-ray showing sacroiliac joint fusion*

Figure 8.6 *X-ray showing cervical spine fusion*

Microbiology Gram stain and culture are normal.

Microscopy No crystals can be seen.

The pathology of the enthesopathy consists of inflammatory infiltration with lymphocytes and plasma cells, at ligament attachments and adjacent to bone erosions. Similar findings are found in sacroiliac joint biopsies and those from peripheral synovitis.

Management

The principles are to relieve pain and stiffness, maintain a maximum range of spinal mobility and avoid the deformity associated with dorsal kyphosis with subsequent hip and knee flexion, which are an attempt to compensate for the dorsal kyphosis. A regular exercise programme and maintenance of good posture are imperative (Table 8.3).

Non-steroidal anti-inflammatory agents and simple analgesics are usually sufficient to relieve symptoms. Amitriptyline can be helpful for nocturnal pain. Local corticosteroid injection is useful for enthesitis. Enteric coated sulfasalazine and methotrexate may benefit the peripheral joint synovitis, but SASP is of only marginal benefit demonstrated in meta-analyses. Anti-TNF therapy has been reported as beneficial, for spinal symptoms as synovitis, but has yet to be subject to appropriate clinical trial.

Although the large joint arthritis is self-limiting, long-term hip disease can lead to secondary osteoarthritis presenting with groin pain that may require surgery. Radiotherapy used extensively in the 1950s is now rarely used because of the ten-fold increase in risk of leukaemia.

Table 8.3 Treatment in ankylosing spondylitis

Education	encourage mobilisation (swimming, walking etc.) join self-help group for regular exercise consider appropriate bed
Physiotherapy	back exercises to maintain posture maintain as much mobility as possible
Axial arthritis	non-steroidal anti-inflammatory agents sulfasalazine
Peripheral synovitis	non-steroidal anti-inflammatory agents sulfasalazine; other disease modifying drugs

Prognosis

The vast majority of patients with ankylosing spondylitis maintain normal employment. Restricted chest movement may predispose to respiratory infection. Systemic complications carry the worst prognosis.

Epidemiology

Prevalence of ankylosing spondylitis is about 1%, with a peak onset of disease in the second and third decade and a male:female ratio of 4:1. Dependent on the locality, an average GP practice of 2,500 will have 250 patients with HLA B27, but only 10 males and 1 female with ankylosing spondylitis.

Referral in ankylosing spondylitis

Patients should be referred for:

- investigation of persistent low back pain;
- treatment with appropriate physiotherapy;
- failure to respond to NSAIDs;
- persistently elevated acute phase response;
- acute eye inflammation;
- cardiac problems;
- cauda-equina syndrome;
- acute episodes of back pain.

REACTIVE ARTHRITIS

The aseptic arthritis triggered by an infectious agent at a site outside the joint is known as a reactive arthritis. These arthritides are now considered as part of the spondyloarthropathies, which includes sexually acquired reactive arthritis (SARA), enteropathically acquired reactive arthritis (EARA), and the enteropathic arthropathies associated with bowel disease such as ulcerative colitis, Crohn's disease, Whipple's disease and post-bypass arthritis. Reiter's syndrome is a triad of non-specific urethritis, conjunctivitis and reactive arthritis, and can arise following urogenital tract or gastro–intestinal tract infection. This was first described in German soldiers recruited during the First World War.

Clinical features

Reactive arthritides are initiated by episodes of bacterial dysentery following Salmonella typhimurium, Shigella flexneri, Shigella dysenteriae,

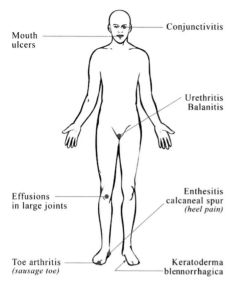

Campylobactera jejuni or Yersinia enterocolitica infection. Alternatively following exposure to chlamydia as a sexually transmitted infection can precipitate these symptoms. Onset of symptoms is typically acute with the symptoms of dysuria and urethritis, conjunctivitis and an inflammatory oligoarthritis, usually affecting large joints of the lower limbs. These can occur up to three months following exposure to the bacterial antigen (Figure 8.7), often when symptoms of the precipitating infection have disappeared. Systemic features of fever and weight loss are not uncommon.

Figure 8.7 *Clinical features of reactive arthritis*

Low back pain and stiffness from sacro-iliitis is present in about 5% of patients at onset, rising to nearly 40% after 15 years. The presence of a reactive arthritis can exist in the absence of conjunctivitis or urethritis, commonly in young men. The arthritis is usually self-limiting with 75% in complete remission at the end of the second year after onset, but it does persist in 15% of cases.

The onset may be insidious but extra symptoms of heel pain (Figure 8.3), tendonitis, fasciitis or the skin rash of keratoderma blennorrhagica on the soles of the feet (Figure 8.8) can assist in making the diagnosis. In addition to the skin lesions, nail dystrophy can also be seen. The conjunctivitis usually subsides spontaneously but iritis can be seen in 10% of cases manifest by the painful blurred vision associated with an irregular semi-reactive pupil and anterior chamber hypopyon. This requires urgent treatment.

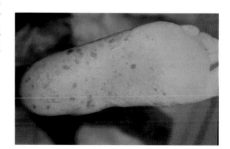

Figure 8.8 *Keratoderma blennorrhagica*

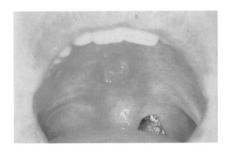

Figure 8.9 *Mouth ulcers*

Urethritis is usually associated with dysuria and sterile discharge. It is more commonly observed in men than women, presumably because urethritis in females may be asymptomatic. Rarely, haemorrhagic cystitis and prostatitis are seen. Oral ulceration (Figure 8.9), pericarditis, aortic insufficiency and transient neurological dysfunction can also be a manifestation of this syndrome.

Investigations

Haematology Raised ESR, with anaemia during acute disease.

Biochemistry Raised CRP which mimics ESR.

Immunology Rheumatoid factor and ANA are universally negative. IgA may be raised. HLA-B27 is more common than in the normal population (50–80%).

X-ray Periarticular osteoporosis erosions and joint space narrowing are rare. Sacro-iliitis enthesitis and periostitis occur (Figure 8.5) where clinical features are found.

Synovial fluid haematology White cell count high ($>10,000\times10^6$/l).

Microbiology Gram stain and culture are normal.

Microscopy No crystals can be seen.

Treatment

Management is mainly symptomatic and supportive (Table 8.5). Non-steroidal anti-inflammatory agents are the mainstay of pain relief, but should be avoided in patients with inflammatory bowel disease. Systemic corticosteroids are rarely required but symptomatic improvement with judicious aspiration of joints and injection of symptomatic enthesopathies will usually control symptoms. Iritis is a medical emergency requiring topical intraocular or systemic corticosteroids. Severe, prolonged, progressive arthritis can warrant disease modifying drug therapy. Urethritis is usually treated with a short course of tetracycline.

Table 8.5 Treatment in reactive arthritis

Education	avoid potential gastrointestinal infections safe sex using condoms
Acute arthritis	aspirate to exclude septic arthritis non-steroidal anti-inflammatory agents simple analgesic inject corticosteroids
Persistent synovitis	sulfasalazine; other disease-modifying drugs

Prevention of reactive arthritis and relapse

Reactive arthritis can be caused by a diverse variety of infectious agents, many of which are never identified. Nevertheless, the number of patients with sexually acquired reactive arthritis has fallen recently, partly due to more effective early treatment of gonococcal urethritis, but presumably also because of the increased use of protective measures during sexual intercourse. Treatment of acute episodes of dysentery would seem appropriate, as would avoidance of potential infected foods.

Epidemiology

An average GP practice of 2,500 will have 250 patients with HLA B27, but this MHC Class I link is less specific for reactive arthritis than it is with AS. A male with B27 runs a 20% risk of developing symptoms after acute gastrointestinal infection. Up to 2% of patients with non-specific urethritis attending the GU medicine clinic have a reactive arthritis, with a similar number developing symptoms following Shigella or Salmonella infection.

Referral in reactive arthritis

Patients should be referred for:

- investigation of acute arthritis;
- persistent synovitis after six months;
- acute iritis;
- exacerbation of gastrointestinal symptoms;
- physiotherapy in axial disease.

ENTERIC ARTHROPATHIES

Reactive arthritis occurs in up to 20% of patients with ulcerative colitis and Crohn's disease. This is usually a mono or symmetrical oligoarthritis with a usual close temporal association between exacerbations of gut and joint symptoms. Knees are the commonest joints involved and attacks are usually self limiting, 50% lasting less than six months and only 20% persisting longer than one year.

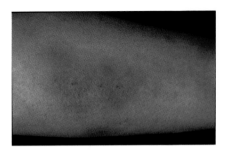

Figure 8.10 *Erythema nodosum*

Enthesopathies, sacroiliitis and spondylitis do occur in patients with inflammatory bowel diseases, but are less common than the peripheral joint synovitis. Erythema nodosum (Figure 8.10) and pyoderma gangrenosum (Figure 6.14) occur in less than 10% of cases of inflammatory bowel disease.

Sub-clinical manifestations of bowel disease can be found in patients with inflammatory arthritis, often whether there is a family history of inflammatory colitis or Crohn's disease.

Treatment is more limiting because NSAIDs can exacerbate colitis. Steroids are used regularly for mono-arthritis, and sulfasalazine can be beneficial for the persistent synovitis and the inflammatory bowel disease.

WHIPPLE'S DISEASE

This is a rare cause of an oligo-arthritis, commonly affecting Caucasian middle-age men with a low-grade fever and weight loss, with anaemia, lymphadenopathy and skin pigmentation. Systemic manifestations include diarrhoea, protein-losing enteropathy and hepato-splenomegally occurs. Patients also develop symptoms of pericarditis, apathy, fits, and meningitis as well as a chronic cough, pleurisy and pulmonary infiltrates on chest X-ray.

Histological features in the synovial membrane mimic those seen in the bowel wall, mainly the presence of large foamy vacuolated macrophages, which contain a small Gram-positive bacillus tropheryma whippelli seen by electron microscopy.

Treatment with tetracycline or penicillin or co-trimoxazole for two weeks or more is rapidly beneficial, but relapse, often with CNS manifestations occur in 30% of cases. These necessitate prolonged treatment.

Lyme disease

Lyme disease is classically characterised by an initial erythematous skin reaction at the site of a tick bite, associated with constitutional symptoms of fatigue, malaise, arthralgia, hepatitis and meningeal irritation and signs of pharyngitis, pleurisy and lymphadenopathy. This immune reaction follows infection with Borrelia burgdorferi, a spirochaete that infects *Ixodes* ticks whose primary host is sheep and deer which subsequently bite human patients. If untreated half the patients develop a mono or oligo large joint arthritis with the knee being the commonest involved. The synovial fluid shows an inflammatory pattern and villous hypertrophy and endarteritis has been seen on synovial biopsy. Neurological involvement is also frequent with meningitis, encephalopathy, radiculitis and cranial neuropathies. Rarely, cardiac manifestations are reported with myocarditis and varying degrees of heart block.

The diagnosis of Borrelia infection rests on the presence of IgM anti-Borrelia antibodies during the acute phase of infection with IgG class detected later in disease. These antibodies can be found in serum, synovial fluid and cerebrospinal fluid. Treatment is with penicillins, tetracyclines and cephalosporins to which Borrelia burgdorferi is usually sensitive.

Rheumatic fever

The classical presentation of rheumatic fever includes a flitting large joint polyarthritis, with involvement of the central nervous system often with chorea and evidence of a carditis and inflammation of the heart valves. These symptoms together with subcutaneous nodules and erythema marginatum represent the major Duckett-Jones criteria for the diagnosis and follow preceding infection with group A streptococci, usually in teenage children. Minor criteria include fever, arthralgias, leucocytosis and raised acute phase response. The diagnosis is confirmed by the presence of evidence of infection with streptocccal infection. Although there is a declining incidence because of antibiotic use for upper respiratory tract infections, there is evidence of increasing virulence in recent studies.

Treatment is hospital-based with aspirin, but in the presence of carditis steroid therapy can be instigated. Penicillin should be started even in the absence of pharyngitis and continued for ten days to eradicate the infection. Prophylaxis with penicillin or erythromycin should be continued until a young adult, and patients should be vaccinated with streptococcal vaccines.

ARTHRITIS DERMATITIS SYNDROME LINKED TO BY-PASS SURGERY

Up to 30% of patients following jejuno-colic by-pass can develop synovitis, often of small joints of the hands and feet in the manner resembling rheumatoid arthritis, starting up to three years post-surgery. Erosive disease is rare, and rheumatoid factor and ANA are negative. The skin lesions associated with this arthropathy occur in up to 80% of cases. Although some of these lesions are vasculitis on biopsy, many have an urticarial or pathovascular aetiology. Treatment is symptomatic.

SARCOIDOSIS

Less than 10% of all cases of systemic sarcoidosis have musculoskeletal problems. The usual presentation to rheumatologists is with acute sarcoidosis with erythema nodosum (Figure 8.10), hilar lymphadenopathy (Figure 8.11) and flitting arthralgias in which case more than 60% of cases have the arthropathy. The prognosis is good and usually only requires symptomatic control with non steroidal anti-inflammatory drugs. Routine investigations demonstrate an elevated acute phase response anaemia and thrombophilia. Leucopaenia is found in 33% of cases and an eosinophilia in a further 25%. However serum calcium is only elevated in 11%. The serum angiotensin converting enzyme is raised in 50-60% of cases.

Chronic synovitis is rare (Figure 8.12) except when the non caseating granulomas seen in synovial biopsies also affects underlying bone when an x-ray may show cysts. In this situation, chest x-ray usually shows pulmonary infiltration with restrictive pulmonary function tests, and systemic corticosteroid therapy may be required to regulate symptom control.

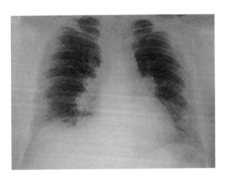

Figure 8.11   *Hilar lymphadenopathy*

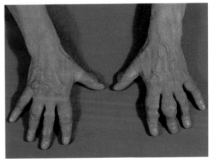

Figure 8.12   *Arthritis of chronic sarcoidosis*

RELAPSING POLYCHONDRITIS

This rare condition characterised by chronic lymphocyte and neutrophil infiltration into cartilage tissues is often found secondary to underlying connective tissue diseases including rheumatoid arthritis and psoriatic arthritis. It predominately affects Caucasian, middle-aged subjects and presents with recurrent painful swellings of external ear (Figure 8.13), nose, and uveitis in the presence of an arthropathy. These attacks are short lived, but repeated episodes produce deformity of nose and ears and joint destruction. Involvement of bronchial cartilage can lead to airway collapse with symptoms of stridor, dyspnoea and dysphonia, with tenderness over thyroid and trachea indicate more extensive disease. Relapses are characterised by a high acute phase response, circulating antibodies

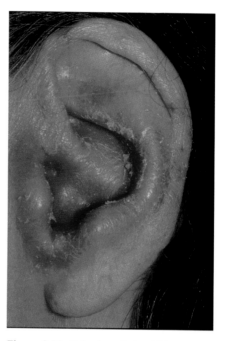

Figure 8.13 *Relapsing polychondritis*

against type II collagen and CT or MRI scan demonstrating the extent of local disease. Treatment is with non steroidal anti-inflammatory drugs, but rarely corticosteroids and immunosuppression are required. Chronic synovitis is rare except when the non-caseating granulomas seen in synovial biopsies also affects underlying bone when an x-ray may show cysts.

chapter 9

Psoriatic arthritis

This is defined as an inflammatory arthritis associated with psoriasis. Psoriatic lesions usually occur over the extensor services, and are associated with nail changes including pitting and onycholysis and hyperkeratosis.

CLINICAL FEATURES

In 15% of cases, the arthritis precedes the skin rash, but there is usually a family history of psoriasis. The psoriatic arthritides are usually rheumatoid factor negative and nodules are absent. The arthritis can be subdivided into five groups (Table 9.1, Figure 9.1)

■ Classical psoriatic arthritis with distal interphalangeal joint in-volvement of hands and feet (Figure 9.2).
■ Symmetrical polyarthritis indistinguishable from rheumatoid but with a negative serology.
■ An asymmetrical pauciarticular arthritis with small joint involvement often with dactylitis (sausage digits).
■ Ankylosing spondylitis pattern with or without peripheral arthritis.
■ Arthritis mutilans (Figure 9.3). A destructive, deforming polyarthritis with loss of joints and periarticular bone structure leading to telescoping of the fingers.

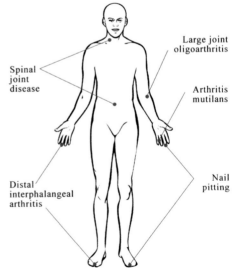

Figure 9.1 *Distribution of psoriatic arthritis*

Table 9.1 Different forms of psoriatic arthritis

Asymmetrical polyarthritis	70%	Proximal joints hands/feet Sausage digits Like reactive arthritis
Ankylosing spondylitis	20%	Can also have features of reactive arthritis
Symmetrical polyarthritis	10%	Similar to rheumatoid arthritis Can have extra-articular features
Distal interphalangeal joints	10%	Dactylitis a common feature Nail changes frequently seen
Arthritis mutilans	5%	Destructive polyarthritis Telescoping of fingers Dissolving bone Spinal ankylosis can be seen

Changes found outwith the joint include conjunctivitis, iritis and episcleritis. These are usually found in association with the ankylosing spondylitis pattern of psoriatic arthritis.

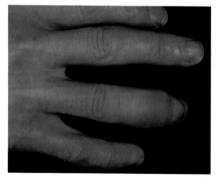

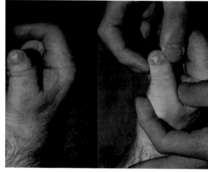

Figure 9.2 *Psoriatic arthritis of distal interphalangeal joint ring finger with nail pitting on the middle finger*

Figure 9.3 *Arthritis mutilans*

INVESTIGATIONS

Haematology
ESR is high with the symmetrical polyarthritis, but otherwise the ESR is usually only moderately raised. Normochromic normocytic anaemia is present.

Immunology
Rheumatoid factor and ANA are predominantly negative.

X-ray
Damage to distal interpha-langeal joints (Figure 9.4), sacroiliac joint, lumbar spine will be involved, dependent on the clinical pattern.

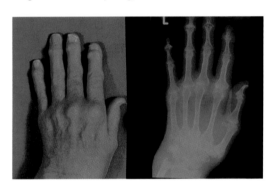

Figure 9.4 *Hand and X-ray showing changes in distal interphalangel joints*

TREATMENT OF PSORIATIC ARTHRITIS

Present management regimes are similar to inflammatory synovitis (Table 9.2). Patient education is of paramount importance together with appropriate physiotherapy to maintain posture in the spondylitis patients and joint mobility in those with peripheral joint disease.

Symptom control with NSAIDs and simple analgesics can be all that is required. However, DMARD therapy with standard agents particularly sulfasalazine, methotrexate and cyclosporin A is beneficial, with the latter two being reported useful for control of psoriasis as well. Hydroxychloroquine has been reported to cause deterioration of skin disease, but is still used. Retinol and photochemotherapy with methylpsoralen that are used primarily for skin disease can also be beneficial in cases where the deterioration of arthritis and skin lesions coincide. Immunosuppressive drugs including azathioprine, and cyclophosphamide are used, as are small doses of oral prednisolone. Intra-articular steroid treatment, rehabilitation, and surgical treatments are used as with other arthritides.

HIV positive individuals can present with deterioration in skin and joint disease following methotrexate therapy producing an erythroderma

Table 9.2 Treatment of psoriatic arthritis

Regular treatment	Education	join appropriate disease group swimming and exercise
Peripheral arthritis	Physiotherapy	maintain range of movement maintain posture and function
	Medical	non steroidal anti-inflammatory drugs sulfasalazine methotrexate penicillamine gold cyclosporin A
	Surgical	joint replacement as required
Axial arthritis	Physiotherapy	maintain appropriate posture
	Medical	non steroidal anti-inflammatory drugs sulfasalazine
Skin lesions	Topical	coal tar creams and shampoos dithranol
	Systemic	psoralens with UV irradiation methotrexate and cyclosporin A

appearance in severe cases. Early studies with hydroxychloroquine showed occasional exacerbation of skin lesions follow treatment, so anti-malarials have not frequently been used, but this view is being challenged recently. Intravenous glucocorticoids are contraindicated as methylprednisolone can exacerbate the skin disease.

Prognosis

This tends to be better than for rheumatoid arthritis but those associated with a poorer prognosis are of younger age and those with extensive skin involvement with psoriasis, and patients with arthritis mutilans. The presence of HLA-B27 correlates with ankylosing spondylitis and the HLA-DR3 and HLA-DR4 are associated with a more erosive disease.

EPIDEMIOLOGY

Psoriatic arthritis affects 10% of patients with psoriasis. In a standard general practitioner's list of 2,500 patients there will be five to 10 patients with psoriatic arthritis.

REFERRAL

Patients should be referred for:

- exclusion of inflammatory synovitis;
- active persistent synovitis (more than three months);
- failure of synovitis to respond to systemic treatment ;
- surgical advice about joint replacement.

chapter 10

Connective tissue diseases

SYSTEMIC LUPUS ERYTHEMATOSUS

Introduction

Systemic lupus erythematosus (SLE) is a classical autoimmune connective tissue disease that affects all medical systems (Figure 10.1) and every race, but

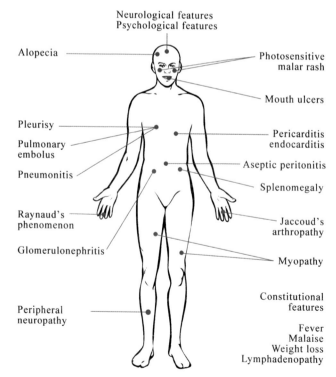

Neurological features
Psychological features

Alopecia

Photosensitive malar rash

Mouth ulcers

Pleurisy

Pericarditis
endocarditis

Pulmonary embolus

Aseptic peritonitis

Pneumonitis

Splenomegaly

Raynaud's phenomenon

Jaccoud's arthropathy

Glomerulonephritis

Myopathy

Peripheral neuropathy

Constitutional features

Fever
Malaise
Weight loss
Lymphadenopathy

Figure 10.1 *Clinical features of SLE*

with different clinical manifestations being more common in each. The common theme is the presence of circulating auto-antibodies and immune complexes that deposit in and around blood vessel walls and induce complement mediated damage in various organs. Deficiency of the early components of the complement pathway is one cause of SLE, but these are extremely rare so in the majority the cause is unknown. Nevertheless, SLE has a multifactorial aetiology with a strong genetic influence in all races that is likely to result from inheritance of more than one gene. Environmental factors are also relevant with the high incidence in pre-menopausal females, the frequent onset during or after pregnancy indicating hormonal factors. Other environmental factors implicated in the aetiology include ultraviolet light, infection and administration of certain drugs.

Although a multifactorial aetiology is recognised, there is profound disturbance of all parts of the immune system with auto-antibody production by B cells, failure to remove circulating immune complexes by the mononuclear phagocytic system, and impaired T cell function. Although there is no unifying hypothesis as to the cause of SLE, auto-antibody production is probably driven by auto-antigens released from dying lymphocytes. Much of the tissue damage probably results from direct action of these antibodies in a type II hypersensitivity (haemolytic anaemia), or by type III hypersensitivity (immune complex mediated glomerulonephritis).

Clinical features

The clinical manifestations of SLE are legion and vary between racial groups and in individual patients. Specific features of SLE are defined by the American College of Rheumatology (Table 10.1) and patients fulfilling four or more criteria have sufficient to make a diagnosis of SLE. However, many features are less specific including fever, malaise and tiredness but all are commonly recognised in these patients. Because of the multisystem involvement symptoms are best described by system.

The skin These are well recognised by virtue of their ease of recognition. The malar rash over the cheeks and bridge of the nose is classical in Caucasian patients (Figure 10.2), and is often worse after ultraviolet light exposure (Figure 10.3), but only occurs in around 50% of cases. Raynaud's phenomenon (Figure 10.4) is present in 30-50%, and can precede the onset of periungual erythema and vasculitis with nail fold or digital infarction. Livido reticularis (Figure 10.5) occur in SLE patients often in association with anti-cardiolipin antibodies and subacute cutaneous lupus (Figure 10.6) in association with antibodies against La (SS-B). Discoid lupus (Figure 10.7)

Table 10.1 American College of Rheumatology: diagnostic criteria for SLE

- Malar rash
- Discoid rash
- Photosensitivity
- Oral ulceration
- Arthritis (two or more joints)
- Serositis (pleurisy or pericarditis)
- Renal disease (+++ or < 0.5gm proteinuria or cellular casts)
- Neurological features (psychosis epilepsy)
- Haematological disorders (haemolytic anaemia, lymphopaenia, thrombocytopaenia)
- Immunological disorders (anti-dsDNA, anti-Sm, lupus anticoagulant)
- Anti-nuclear antibody

The diagnosis is made when four or more features are present simultaneously or serially

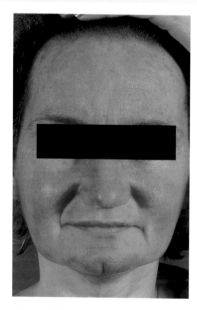

Figure 10.2 *Facial rash*

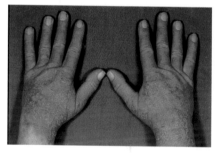

Figure 10.3 *Photosensitivity*

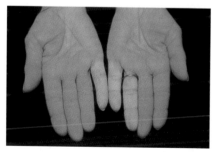

Figure 10.4 *Raynaud's phenomenon*

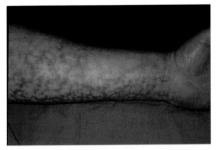

Figure 10.5 *Livido reticularis*

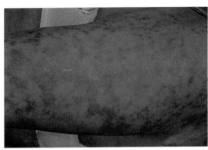

Figure 10.6 *Subacute cutaneous lupus*

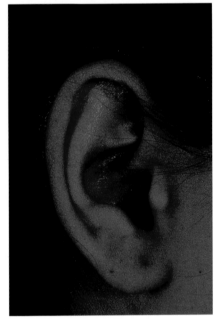

Figure 10.7 *Discoid lupus*

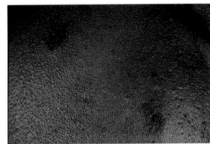

Figure 10.8 *Follicular plugging*

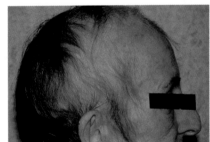

Figure 10.9 *Alopecia*

can occur in isolation and is more common in pigmented skin, and similarly follicular plugging (Figure 10.8) is also more common in non-Caucasians. Oral ulcers occur commonly, but nasal and vaginal ulcers are also well recognised in SLE. Alopecia can lead to quite marked hair loss and is seen in over 50% of cases (Figure 10.9).

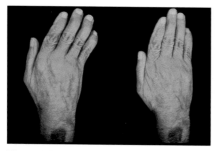

Figure 10.10 *The correctable deformity of Jaccoud's arthropathy*

The joints Arthralgia is common, occurring in around 90% of cases, but true synovitis is less frequent (around 50%), and is present in a polyarticular distribution. Although joint deformity is unusual when

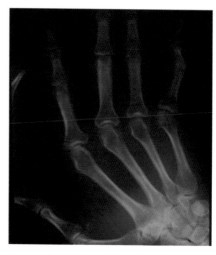

Figure 10.11 *X-ray of Jaccoud's arthropathy*

present it is usually correctable (in contrast to rheumatic arthritis) and is named after Jaccoud (Figure 10.10). Erosive changes on x-ray are minimal if present at all (Figure 10.11), with some of the features of pain and stiffness being attributed to tenosynovitis rather than arthritis. Myalgias are not uncommon but true myositis is less frequent. Musculoskeletal complications of SLE include tendon rupture and avascular necrosis, both of which are probably at least in part due to corticosteroid therapy.

The kidneys Glomerulonephritis (Figure 10.12) develops in approximately 50% of SLE patients with varying histological features resulting from immune complex deposition within glomeruli (Figure 10.13). The presence

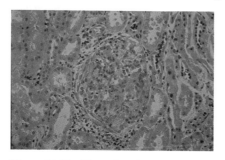

Figure 10.12 *Glomerulonephritis*

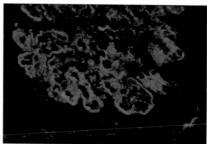

Figure 10.13 *Immunofluorescence of glomerulonephritis*

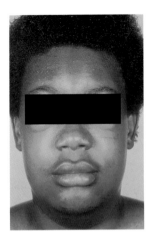

Figure 10.14 *Nephrotic syndrome*

of hypertension, proteinuria, and renal failure with casts in the urine is indicative of nephritis that can respond well to high dose corticosteroids and cyclophosphamide. Nephrotic syndrome occurs when oedema affecting the periphery but also the face (Figure 10.14) results from severe leakage of albumin from damaged glomeruli. Renal tubular disease with renal tubular acidosis may be present but is usually asymptomatic.

The lungs Recurrent pleurisy and pleural effusion (an exudate) are common and pulmonary emboli secondary to clotting disorders need to be excluded. Pneumonitis can occur in association with fever, dyspnoea in the absence of infection, and lung fibrosis can also occur with restrictive lung function tests indicating impairment of ventilation and perfusion. Shrinking lung syndrome manifests as increasing shortness of breath with progressive loss of lung volume. Pulmonary hypertension can result from lung damage with the poor prognosis associated with this manifestation.

The heart Serositis can also affect the pericardium. Myocarditis is rare, but can produce tachycardia, arrhythmias and cardiac failure often during disease exacerbations with associated ECG abnormalities. Valvular involvement with Libman Sachs endocarditis is rare, but systolic murmers may be detected because of the hyperdynamic circulation. The commonest cardiac feature of SLE at the turn of the millenium is coronary vascular involvement with arteriosclerotic disease attributed to immune complex damage and corticosteroid use.

The central nervous system The central nervous system involvement is an important cause of morbidity. The majority of symptoms, however, are mild with headache, psychosis and epilepsy being the most common. Meninges spinal cord or peripheral nerves can be affected producing a variety of features including peripheral neuropathy, transverse myelitis, hemiplegia severe psychosis, many of which can change dependent upon disease activity. Irreversible dementia may also occur possibly due to a combination of direct neuronal damage and arteriosclerosis.

The lymphoid and haemopoietic system Lymphadenopathy occurs in up to 50% of cases with non-specific inflammatory changes seen on biopsy. Involvement of haemopoietic system includes anaemia of chronic disease, or from haemolysis. Clotting abnormalities associated with anti-phospholipid antibodies and the lupus anticoagulant are present in about 25% of cases. Leucopenia, and particularly lymphopenia are frequent but neutropaenia is rarer, probably secondary to antibodies directed against the neutrophil cell membrane encouraging their removal from the circulation. Thrombocytopenia is rare and has a similar aetiology, but only rarely leads to sufficiently low levels leading to purpura (Figure 10.10) and requiring corticosteroids or gamma globulin to prevent serious damage from blood loss.

The eyes Many patients develop secondary Sjögren's syndrome, usually after life-long involvement with SLE but episcleritis and optic neuritis can also be found. Retinal vasculitis with cotton wool spots can be seen during acute disease exacerbation and can rarely cause retinal infarction.

The anti-phospholipid syndrome (APLS) APLS can occur in association with SLE and other connective tissue diseases, but can be seen in isolation in their absence. The APLS is characterised by vascular thrombosis, thrombocytopenia and recurrent spontaneous miscarriage. Circulating antibodies against phospholipids, particularly cardiolipin are present, and lupus anticoagulant is positive in some cases. Treatment is aimed at prevention of thrombosis with aspirin or anticoagulation with warfarin. Catastrophic anti-phospholipid syndrome can occur with widespread intravascular thrombosis, precipitating fever, malaise and symptoms of arterial and venous structure. Often the INR needs to be between 3.0 and 4.0 to reduce the frequency of thromboses. Maintainance of good anticoagulant control with aspirin and/or heparin during pregnancy increases the likelyhood of a foetus developing to term.

Investigations

Haematology ESR is raised. Haemoglobin is low/normal: haemolytic or B12 or iron deficient. White cell count is low with lymphopaenia and/or neutropaenia and/or thrombocytopaenia.

Biochemistry Urea/creatinine level is raised in glomerular involvement. There is impaired creatinine clearance and proteinuria if glomerular involvement. There may be abnormal liver function rarely and raised creatine kinase in myositis.

Immunology Antinuclear antibodies are virtually always positive (Figure 10.15), usually with a homogeneous pattern (anti-DNA antibodies) or a

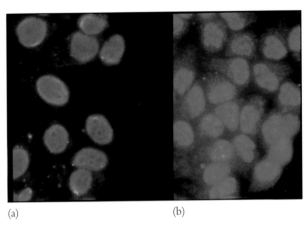

Figure 10.15 *Antinuclear antibodies*
(a) *homogeneous pattern*
(b) *speckled pattern*

(a)   (b)

speckled pattern (antibodies against RNA binding proteins). Rheumatoid factor may be positive.

X-ray Non erosive changes will be shown unless severe arthritis (Figure 10.11).

Synovial fluid haematology White cell count will be >3,000x10^6/l.

Microbiology Gram stain and culture are normal.

Specialist investigations

The antinuclear antibody screening test for SLE is usually positive (around 97% of cases). Anti-double stranded DNA antibodies (45%) are SLE specific and vary with disease activity. Antibodies against extractable nuclear antigens (RNA binding proteins—Sm, RNP, Ro and La) are common (around 60% of cases). Rheumatoid factor may be positive in up to 50% of cases. Serum complement factor 4 (C4) is usually low—a genetic predisposition. Sequential measurement of total C3 and C4 fall during active disease. Complement breakdown products rise during active disease.

Clotting studies may show lupus anticoagulant (30% of cases). Prolonged clotting times are not corrected by the addition of normal serum. Anti-cardiolipin antibodies are present (50% of cases).

MRI and CT scans can show abnormalities in the presence of cerebral lupus. EMG, MRI and muscle biopsy are helpful in presence of myositis (qv). Renal biopsy (Figures 10.11, 10.12) can be useful in demonstrating glomerulonephritis, graded according to active and chronic criteria to guide underlined treatment.

Table 10.2 Treatment of systemic lupus erythematosus

Supportive measures
- Patient education is of paramount importance.
- Local lupus groups can be particularly helpful in providing support.
- Specific treatment with physiotherapy and occupational therapy useful if arthritis is a feature.

Drug treatment
- Skin disease: sunscreens and topical corticosteroids; hydroxychloroquine.
- Joint pain: non-steroidal anti-inflammatory agents; low dose amitriptyline. May require systemic steroids.
- Renal disease: systemic corticosteroids and immunosupression.
- Cerebral disease: systemic corticosteroids and immunosupression.
- Intravenous cyclophosphamide reduces development of renal failure .
- Azathioprine is a useful steroid sparing agent.
- Methotrexate and cyclosporin have been used to good effect but remain under study.
- Long term corticosteroid use should be accompanied by therapy to prevent osteoporosis.
- Low dose aspirin is indicated in patients with anti-phospholipid syndrome.
- Anticoagulation with warfarin is necessary if serious thrombotic events occur.

Treatment of systemic lupus erythematosus

There is no cure for SLE so the primary object of treatment is to reduce symptoms. This may be attained using simple analgesics or anti-inflammatory drugs alone, but hydroxychloroquine is useful for skin and joint symptoms. Immunosupression may be required for the more severe life-threatening disorders including renal and cerebral manifestations (Table 10.2)

The disease naturally undergoes flares and remissions, with flares characterised by increase in symptoms (rarely do new ones develop). Aggressive therapy may be needed including steroids and cyclophosphamide to regulate symptoms. Recently intravenous immunoglobulin has been advocated; this has yet to be evaluated properly but is useful particularly for idiopathic thrombocytopaenic purpura (ITP). Methotrexate and cyclosporin have also been advocated but again these need appropriate clinical trials to confirm their efficacy. Severe symptoms might necessitate bone marrow transplantation.

Treatment of neonatal lupus

Skin rash disappears within three months as maternal antibodies are removed from the circulation, and may require topical steroid therapy.

Treatment of congenital heart block is more complex as 75% of at risk mothers produce a normal foetus. Recommendations at present are for regular foetal monitoring for heart rate in at risk patients with circulating anti-La antibodies, and the use of plasmaphoresis and dexamethasone upon detection of the abnormal heart rate. Cardiac pacemaker may be necessary early post-partum but may not be required until later childhood.

Pregnancy in systemic lupus erythematosus

Pregnancy is no longer contraindicated in SLE provided the disease is stable. The possible problems are set out in Table 10.3. Previous active disease may have necessitated treatment with cyclophosphamide that may precipitate ovarian or testicular failure. Problems for the mother include disease exacer-

---

Table 10.3 Pregnancy in SLE and related diseases

- Prolonged use of cyclophosphamide is a significant cause of ovarian or testicular failure.
- Pregnancy is not contraindicated provided the SLE disease is stable.
- Problems are more likely in patients with active renal and cerebral disease.
- Hydroxychloroquine causes VIIIth nerve damage especially during the first trimester.
- Prednisolone is not contraindicated during pregnancy.
- Non steroidal anti-inflammatory drugs can cross the placenta.
- Complications of pregnancy for the mother:
  - exacerbation of SLE: this is unusual;
  - skin and joint complications can respond to simple analgesics and local measures;
  - renal and cerebral complications may necessitate immunosupression;
  - spontaneous abortion may be caused by intra-placental clotting linked with anti-cardiolipin antibodies and lupus anticoagulant.

Complications of pregnancy for the foetus:
  - antibodies cross the placenta and can cause local damage;
  - anti-La antibodies are linked with neonatal cardiac damage;
  - cardiac damage can be localised to Bundle of His or be more extensive;
  - the facial rash of neonatal SLE clears as maternal antibodies disappear.

bation that is more likely to occur if the disease is active. Spontaneous abortion occurs more regularly with all its complications, particularly those with anti-phopholipid antibodies. Complications of neonatal involvement secondary to trans-placental passage of maternal antibodies have been described above.

Prognosis

Complete remission in SLE is rare, but the ten-year survival figures are now higher than 90% because less severe cases are diagnosed, but also because of better and more directed treatment. Infection, renal failure and cerebral lupus remain the common causes of death. Complications of corticosteroids can cause considerable morbidity such as cardiovascular disease, avascular necrosis of the hip, hypertension and diabetes.

Epidemiology

SLE is probably more common than realised, but clinical heterogeneity makes those with milder disease less likely to be diagnosed. In some studies as many as 1 in 250 of the Afro-Caribbean population are affected, but this falls to 1 in 1,000 in the Oriental population and to 1 in 4,500 in the Caucasian. It is therefore likely that one or two patients exist in the average GP practice. It usually, but not exclusively, affects those of childbearing age (25-45); 90% are female, and SLE is more common in urban populations. There is a strong genetic tendency with a high incidence in identical twins and a higher prevalence in family members of the probands. In the Caucasian patients there is a strong association with the HLA haplotype A1 B8 DR3 DQ2 that is associated with the null allele at the C4 locus. However SLE probably has a polygenic aetiology with each clinical feature being dictated by different combinations of genes.

Referral in connective tissue diseases

Patients should be referred for:
- investigation of acute arthritis;
- investigation of skin rashes;
- investigation of myalgias;
- investigation of systemic features;
- characterisation of connective tissue disease;
- persistent synovitis after six months;
- investigation of renal disease;
- treatment of any features of SLE;
- treatment during pregnancy.

SYSTEMIC SCLEROSIS

Scleroderma

This is a multi-system group of disorders of connective tissue characterised by inflammation, fibrosis and degenerative changes in the skin (Table 10.4). Systemic involvement with internal organ damage can involve the gastrointestinal tract, cardiac tissue, lung and kidney and has a sinister association. Raynaud's phenomenon is an almost universal feature in the systemic sclerosis syndromes (Figure 10.16).

The aetiology remains unknown; a genetic predisposition is possible, but environmental factors including vinyl chloride, toxic oils contaminating rapeseed oil and L-tryptophan have been implicated in the development of the spectrum of scleroderma disease. The disease affects primarily females with an annual incidence of 12 per million.

Table 10.4 Systemic sclerosis (SS) syndromes

Raynaud's phenomenon	localised vascular spasm vasoconstriction, pallor, cyanosis, parasthesiae
Morphoea	localised patch of thickened skin Rarely develops into systemic forms
Limited cutaneous SS	Longstanding Raynaud's phenomenon finger and forearm involvement, digits can ulcerate and calcify telangectasia, trigeminal neuralgia antibodies against centromere in 75% of cases late onset pulmonary hypertension
Diffuse cutaneous SS	Late onset Raynaud's phenomenon with new skin changes early lung involvement often with renal failure gastrointestinal and cardiac involvement skin disease in fingers and spreads proximally microstomia and beaked nose appearance antibodies against nucleolus (topoisomerase 1 or Scl 70)

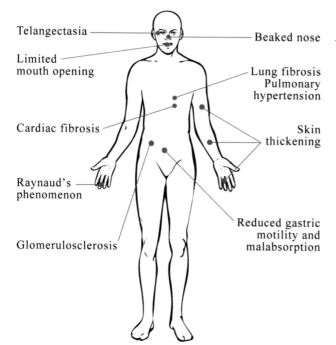

Telangectasia

Limited
mouth opening

Cardiac fibrosis

Raynaud's
phenomenon

Glomerulosclerosis

Beaked nose

Lung fibrosis
Pulmonary
hypertension

Skin
thickening

Reduced gastric
motility and
malabsorption

Figure 10.16 *Clinical features of systemic sclerosis syndromes*

Skin changes

Raynaud's phenomenon (Figure 10.4) is common in 5% of the population commonly young underweight females. Smoking is a common factor and should be discouraged. Usually it is not associated with any underlying disease, but can cause significant symptoms and may need vasodilators to reduce symptoms. Raynaud's phenomenon is the commonest first sign of scleroderma being present in over 90% of cases. The early lesion is one of vascular damage to small arteries, arterioles and capillaries with intimal damage, increasing vascular permeability. Local release of cytokines, which activate fibroblasts and increase collagen and fibronectin synthesis occurs in sites of skin and internal organ involvement.

The skin develops from a well indurated non-pitting swelling of the digits (sausage fingers, Figure 10.17) to skin atrophy (Figure 10.18) with a shiny, leathery and thickened appearance (sclerodactyly) that is frequently associated with ulceration of the fingertips (Figure 10.19), which may calcify. Pigment changes are frequent with either hyper or hypopigmentation occurring (Figure 10.18). As the disease progresses, skin tightening may occur over

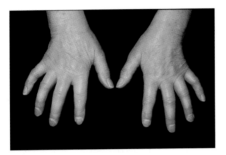

Figure 10.17 *Sausage fingers*

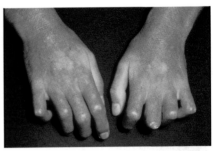

Figure 10.18 *Fixed flexion deformitis*

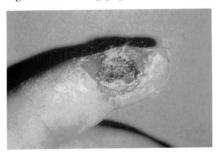

Figure 10.19 *Digital ischeamia*

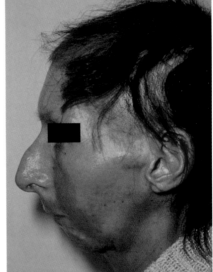

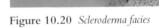

Figure 10.21 *Limited mouth opening*

Figure 10.20 *Scleroderma facies*

bony prominences producing flexion contractures and increasing the risk of skin trauma at these sites. The face may become taught and mask-like with a beak nose and prognathism (Figure 10.20) cause some difficulty in opening the mouth (Figure 10.21) and associated problems with dentition.

Telangectasia (Figure 10.22) are common on the face and upper limbs, and are more common in the limited forms of disease. Nailfold changes occur with both limited and systemic forms with deformed nailfold capillaries that progress to capillary atrophy.

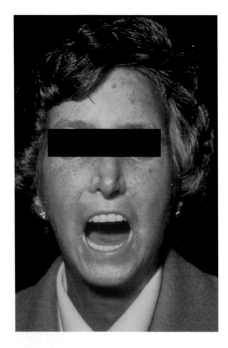

Gastrointestinal tract

Involvement of the gastrointestinal tract with systemic forms of systemic sclerosis can produce limited peristalsis of the oesophagus detected on barium swallowing with symptoms of heartburn, reflux and difficulty of swallowing. Aspiration pneumonia from dilated oesophageal tract can occasionally occur. Dilatation on small segments of large and small bowel can cause intermittent abdominal pain, constipation and obstruction. Malabsorption can occur secondary to bacterial overgrowth. Many patients develop symptoms of Sjögren's syndrome, and some of primary biliary cirrhosis.

Figure 10.22 *Telangectasia*

Lung involvement

Pulmonary fibrosis that classically affects the lower lobes can be seen on fine cut CT scan (Figure 10.23) causing defects in chest expansion and also in gas transfer. Pulmonary function tests show a progressive restrictive pattern. Pulmonary hypertension can result either from primary vascular disease or secondary to lung fibrosis.

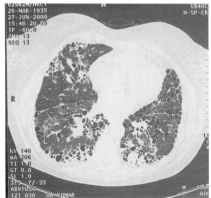

Figure 10.23 *CT scan showing lung fibrosis*

Heart involvement

Cardiac involvement occurs with myocardial fibrosis that can lead to arrhythmias and conduction defects. Pericarditis is recorded, but rarely causes significant symptoms, but pulmonary hypertension can cause secondary right ventricular damage and failure.

Renal involvement

Renal involvement due to arterial intimal proliferation and fibrinoid necrosis causes renal failure and can precipitate systemic hypertension.

Investigations

Haematology Normochromic normocytic anaemia is seen usually with normal ESR.

Biochemistry Renal function, liver function may be abnormal if affected.

Immunology ANA is positive in approximately 50% of patients with a nucleolar (Figure 10.24) or speckled staining pattern. Antibodies to Scl–70 are found in patients with systemic disease. Rheumatoid factor is present in 30% of cases.

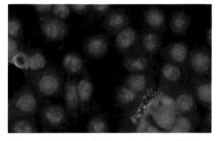

Histology Lung biopsy can show cellular infiltration with or without fibrosis. Skin biopsy shows loss of

Figure 10.24 *Nucleolar antinuclear antibodies*

sweat glands and hair follicles and fibrosis in the dermal tissues. Renal biopsy shows fibrinoid necrosis and intimal changes.

Imaging Chest x-ray and fine cut CT scan will show lung fibrosis and quantify extent. Hand x-rays show fixed flexion deformities, calcium deposits at finger tips. Fine cut CT scan will demonstrate lung fibrosis. Barium studies show oesophageal dilatation and delayed gastric emptying.

Management

There is no specific drug therapy that has proved to be effective in preventing progression of systemic sclerosis. Symptomatic treatment includes protection from the cold with heated gloves and socks, appropriate clothing and non steroidal anti-inflammatory agents where appropriate. Treatment of Raynaud's phenomenon is by avoiding vasoconstricting drugs and with oral nifedepine and intravenous prostacyclin infusions as vasodilators. Angiotensin converting enzyme inhibitors are useful in renal crisis and accelerated hypertension. Corticosteroids may be useful if there is associated myositis and significant arthritis. Penicillamine has been beneficial in some cases attributed to its ability to reduce collagen cross-linking.

Table 10.5 Management of systemic sclerosis	
Education	Self help groups
	Advice on clothing
	Avoidance of cold and vasoconstricting drugs
	Heated gloves and socks
	Physiotherapy for joint contractures
Raynaud's phenomenon	Vasodilators, inositol nicotinate, nifedepine and prostacycline infusions
Arthritis	Non steroidal anti-inflammatory drugs
Hypertension	ACE inhibitors
Cardiac problems	Anti-arrhythmic drugs
	Diuretics
Myositis	Corticosteroids
Gastrointestinal problems	Antacids
	Drugs to control motility
	Antibiotics to prevent bacterial overgrowth

Prognosis

The prognosis in diffuse systemic sclerosis appears to be relentless with widespread skin involvement and renal, cardiac or respiratory disease resulting in an overall five-year survival of 70%. In the presence of significant pulmonary hypertension, mortality is 90% at the end of one year. With this in mind, recent studies have suggested that bone marrow transplantation might be indicated, but studies in this area are limited with a high mortality.

SCLERODERMA AND RELATED SYNDROMES

Limited cutaneous scleroderma

This form of scleroderma initially presents with Raynaud's phenomenon, usually for many years without any skin changes initially. However skin involvement is usually limited to the hands, but can involve the forearms and only rarely more centrally. Skin is tight, waxy and tethered producing flexion deformities in the fingers. Painful digital ulcers which can calcify

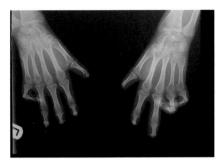

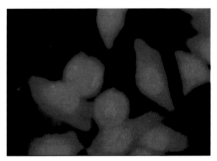

Figure 10.25 *Subcutaneous calcinosis on hand X-ray*

Figure 10.26 *Anti-centromere antinuclear antibodies*

(Figure 10.25) and telangiectasia (Figure 10.22) may occur with dilated nailfold capillaries seen. Oesophageal symptoms can become more severe and patients gradually develop pulmonary hypertension or progressive pulmonary interstitial lung disease. This syndrome used to be known by the acronym CREST (Calcinosis, Raynaud's phenomenon, Esophageal involvement, Sclerodactyly and Telangiectasia). Prognosis in this limited disease is less severe than the diffuse scleroderma, and many patients have antibodies against centromere in their circulation (Figure 10.26).

Morphoea

Linear scleroderma or morphoea consists of well demarcated pale undulated lesions of the skin and subcutaneous tissues can be found mimicking scleroderma. Serological findings rarely show abnormalities, and systemic features are unusual. These forms of this disorder are commonly seen in children and adolescents.

Eosinophilic fasciitis

This is a scleroderma-like condition characterised by pain and swelling and tenderness in the hands, arms and feet. Carpal tunnel compression can be an early feature and symptoms can follow abnormal exercise. Eosinophilia and hyperglobulinaemia are common abnormalities and diagnosis is confirmed by deep skin biopsy that must be deep to show the fascia where eosinophils can be seen infiltrating into the subcutaneous fascia. Eosinophilic fasciitis usually responds to corticosteroids.

POLYMYOSITIS AND DERMATOMYOSITIS

These are autoimmune diseases characterised primarily by inflammation in skeletal muscle. Polymyositis alone represents 40% of cases, but in 15% concomitant skin involvement (dermatomyositis) occurs with the myositis. While either can be secondary to connective tissue diseases in approximately 15% of all cases, polymyositis or dermatomyositis usually occur in isolation. In the elderly (10%) there is a link with underlying malignancy, but although viruses have been implicated as an aetiological agent, none have been proven to be involved.

Polymyositis and dermatomyositis are more common in women with a 3:1 ratio, and a peak incidence between 30-50 with a probable genetic involvement to this disorder linked to HLA-B8 DR3. 10% of all cases are in children where no link with malignant disease is recognised

Clinical features

Polymyositis is usually characterised by gradual onset of proximal painful muscle weakness, particularly affecting the shoulder and pelvic girdles. With weakness and tenderness patients have difficulty in rising from a chair and raising hands above the head. Internal involvement of pharyngeal, laryngeal and respiratory muscles can lead to dysphagia and respiratory failure, necessitating ventilation. There is often associated mild arthralgia or inflammatory arthritis, Raynaud's phenomenon and erythema, some rashes on the elbows and knuckles may be seen.

In adult dermatomyositis, muscle weakness is accompanied by periorbital oedema and a characteristic heliotrope (violet) rash on the upper eyelids (Figure 10.27). A similar coloured rash on the knuckles is termed Gottron's papules (Figure 10.28). There may

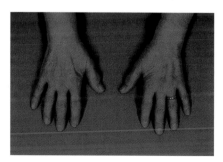

Figure 10.27 *Heliotrope rash*   Figure 10.28 *Gottron's papules*

be a significant arthritis or photosensitive element to the facial skin rash (Figure 10.2), or sclerodactyly (Figure 10.17) and Raynaud's phenomenon (Figure 10.4) raising the possible diagnosis of rheumatoid arthritis, systemic lupus erythematosus or systemic sclerosis, with which there are associations.

Inflammatory myopathies associated with malignancy are uncommon before the age of 40, and are associated with ovarian, gastric and nasopharyngeal carcinomas. Symptoms are usually insidious and in some instances the carcinoma may not become apparent for up to three years. Resection of the tumour can be associated with symptom remission.

Childhood dermatomyositis commonly affects children between the ages of 10 to 20 with muscle weakness and pain and the rashes associated with dermatomyositis. Muscle atrophy and contractures are seen with subcutaneous calcification which can be widespread and severe.

Differential diagnosis
Myasthenia gravis or polymyalgia rheumatica.

Investigations
Haematology Normochromic normocytic anaemia is seen with raised ESR in 50% of cases.

Biochemistry Muscle enzymes, CPK and aldolase are raised, and CRP elevated.

Immunology Antibodies against Jo-1 (tRNA synthetase) are positive in 50% of cases. Rheumatoid factor is present in 50% of cases.

Imaging MRI shows areas of increased water in the inflamed muscle (Figure 10.29).

Histology Inflammatory infiltrate is seen with lymphocytes invading into muscle fibres and centrally placed nuclei in skeletal muscle fibres (Figure 10.30). There is muscle fibre degeneration and regeneration. Antibody staining reveals upregulation of MHC Class I.

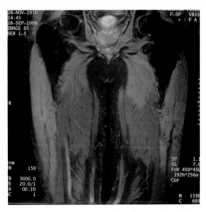

Figure 10.29 *MRI of thigh muscles showing oedema in inflamed vastus lateralis muscle*

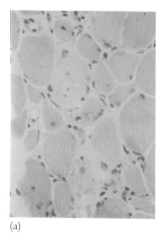
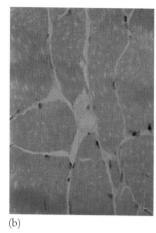

Figure 10.30 *Muscle biopsy in myositis (a) compared to normal sample (b)*

(a)   (b)

EMG There are spontaneous fibrillation and polyphasic action potentials, and repetitive potentials on stimulation of the nerve activating the muscle.

Treatment

Prednisolone in high dose (1mg/kg) induces clinical remission. Creatine kinase level can be followed to monitor clinical improvement. Steroid dose can then be reduced whilst monitoring the whole strength of serum enzyme levels. Immunosuppressive therapy may be required if the steroid response is limited. Physiotherapy and appropriate exercise regimes should help. Azathioprine and methotrexate may be required to help keep the steroid dose to an acceptable minimum. Patients that receive this need protection for osteoporosis whilst on steroids. Recent studies show a benefit of intravenous immunoglobulin.

Prognosis

This is related to whether or not there is an underlying malignancy. In the absence thereof, prognosis is usually good provided acute episode of myositis can be suppressed.

DRUG-INDUCED CONNECTIVE TISSUE DISEASES

Various drugs can precipitate a clinical syndrome similar to SLE. Classically hydrallazine, isoniazid and procainamide have been linked with development of drug-induced SLE (DISLE), but disease modifying drugs for rhuematoid arthritis including sulfasalazine, penicillamine and possibly anti-TNF therapy can have similar effects. Antihypertensives such as beta blockers, methyldopa and ACE inhibitors, and anti-epileptics such as phenytoin hydantoin and primidone and the oestrogen-containing oral contraceptives have also been implicated.

The commonest symptoms of DISLE include arthralgias, skin rashes and an elevated ESR occurring some months after exposure, but serositis lymphadenopathy and hepatosplenomegaly are also reported. The more severe spectrum of SLE, namely renal and cerebral disease, is not usual in DISLE.

Antibodies in DISLE are narrower in profile with antibodies against double stranded DNA and extractable nuclear antigens being rarer while those against RNA, histones and single stranded DNA being more common.

Drug-induced myositis is also a feature of various anti-rheumatic drugs including NSAIDs, and penicillamine and recently with the stain based lipid lowering agents. Myopathies in the absence of inflammation can follow therapy with hydroxychloroquine and colchicine, but also can be seen in patients on lithium clofibrate and amphoteracin treatment.

Drug-induced scleroderma has been reported after treatment with penicillamine, bleomycin and carbidopa, and is also seen following exposure to cocaine.

SJÖGREN'S SYNDROME

Introduction

Sjögren described the syndrome of dry eyes (keratoconjunctivitis sicca), dry mouth (xerostomia) caused by destruction of exocrine glands occuring in the presence of a polyarthritis.

Primary Sjögren's syndrome occurs in isolation, usually in females between the ages of 30 to 50. Often there is major salivary gland enlargement (Figure 10.31) that can be mistaken for mumps or obstruction of the salivary gland ducts because of stones. In secondary Sjögren's syndrome, the symptoms arise in association with a longstanding

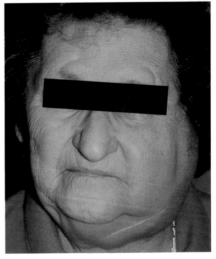

Figure 10.31 *Salivary gland swelling*

underlying connective tissue disease. The commonest of these is rheumatoid arthritis where after ten years most patients have significant ocular and oral symptoms. However, secondary Sjögren's syndrome is also recognised in systemic sclerosis, systemic lupus erythematosus, polymyositis and autoimmune liver disease where erosive arthritis is rarely so prominent a feature.

Pathogenesis

The impaired salivary and lacrimal gland function results from replacement of the normal gland structure with infiltrating CD4+ve memory lymphocytes that is detected on minor salivary gland biopsy (Figure 10.32). In primary Sjögren's syndrome antibodies with a speckled pattern (Figure 10.15) are found. Antibodies against the RNA binding proteins Ro and La are found in 70% and 50% of patients respectively and rheumatoid factor is also commonly detected (in around 90% of cases), and there is a strong genetic link with the autoimmune haplotype HLA A1 B8 DR3.

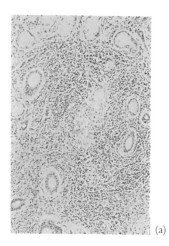
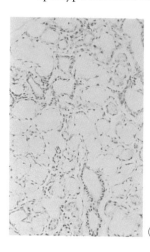

(a) (b)

Figure 10.32 *Salivary gland histology in* (a) *Sjögren's syndrome and* (b) *in a normal biopsy*

Local clinical features

The pathology in primary Sjögren's syndrome leads to destruction of exocrine gland function. Hence symptoms of dryness of the eyes, with a gritty sensation with pain and an itch are common and when severe the keratoconjunctivitis can cause blurred vision and less commonly double vision because the dry cornea sticks to the eyelids. Equally, oral dryness causes severe dental problems with caries and periodontitis (Figure 10.33). The dry skin in Sjögren's syndrome frequently itches and is a cause of

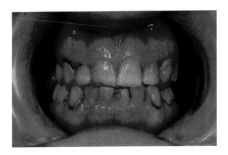

discomfort, and vaginal dryness caused by lack of lubrication can be a significant problem with dyspareunia.

Figure 10.33 *Poor dentition in Sjögren's syndrome*

Systemic clinical features

These are charaterised in Figure 10.34 and Table 10.6. Impaired exocrine gland function also leads to gastrointestinal problems leading to dry mouth with angular stomatitis and oral ulcers. Involvement of the gastrointestinal tract can result in dysphagia and rarely acute or chronic pancreatitis.

Renal involvement includes renal tubular acidosis, and more rarely glomerulonephritis (10% of cases) when some symptoms of Sjögren's syndrome overlap with a diagnosis of SLE.

Neurological involvement can occur either in the CNS or with peripheral neuropathies secondary to vasculitis involving the vasa nervorum. Vasculitis affecting the small blood vessels in the skin occurs in 20% of cases producing a microscopic erythematous rash (Figure 10.35).

Associated systemic features can lead to arthralgia with a non-erosive polyarthritis, much as seen in SLE. Pulmonary involvement can produce lung fibrosis and impaired diffusion defects on pulmonary

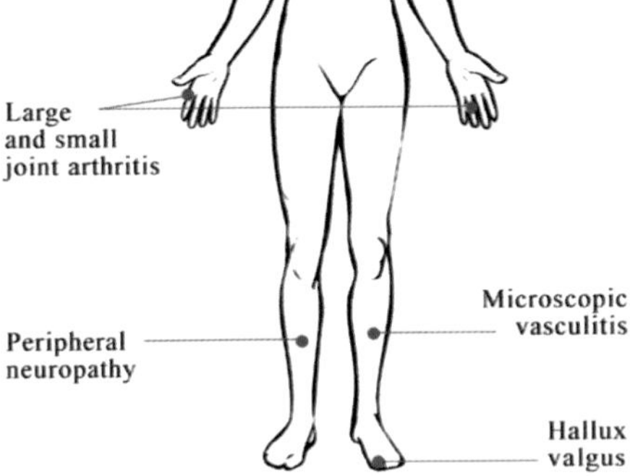

Dry eyes

Dry mouth

Thyroid dysfunction

Lung fibrosis

Large and small joint arthritis

Peripheral neuropathy

Microscopic vasculitis

Hallux valgus

Figure 10.34 *Clinical features of Sjögren's syndrome*

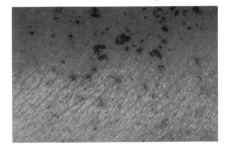

Figure 10.35 *Purpuric vasculitis*

Table 10.6 Features of Sjögren's syndrome

Primary Sjögren's syndrome

- Dry eyes and dry mouth
- Salivary gland enlargement
- Arthritis (usually non or minimally erosive)

- Anaemia, leukopaenia, thrombocytopaenia
- Lymphadenopathy (rarely malignancy)
- Hyperglobulinaemic purpura with vasculitis
- Fibrosing, alveolitis, myositis
- Glomerulonephritis and renal tubular acidosis

- Antinuclear antibody
- Antibodies against Ro and La
- Rheumatoid factor
- Other auto-antibodies

Secondary Sjögren's syndrome

- Dry mouth and dry eyes
- Usually secondary to underlying connective tissue disease
- At least 10% with rheumatoid arthritis
- Rheumatoid factor
- Antinuclear antibodies

function tests. Other autoimmune diseases are also more common including thyroid dysfunction, primary biliary cirrhosis and other autoimmune liver diseases.

There is an increased incidence of non-Hodgkin's B-cell lymphoma that occurs in the salivary glands.

Local investigations

The diagnosis is assessed by using a standard filter paper placed on the lower eyelid. The demonstration of a dry Schirmer's test after ten minutes is positive. Alternatively, positive Rose Bengal staining shows the presence of keratitis that also confirms a diagnosis of Sjögren's syndrome. Impaired salivary flow can also be shown in patients with xerostomia.

Other investigations

Haematology There is low haemoglobin, reduced white cell and platelet count.

Biochemistry Renal function may show tubular acidosis with low bicarbonate, with raised urea and creatinine if glomerular involvement. Liver function tests may be abnormal, with elevated gamma globulins.

Immunology Rheumatoid factor will be present in 90% of cases, with antibodies against Ro (SS-A) and La (SS-B) and antibodies against smooth muscle.

Imaging Radiography will show either no erosions or very small punched out lesions.

Histology There is inflammatory cell infiltrate into the salivary gland.

Predisposition to other disorders

Antibodies against La can cross the placenta and produce congenital foetal heart block, but this occurs most commonly in the first trimester of pregnancy. It occurs in around 5% of patients with circulating anti-La antibodies and 20% of those that have had a previously affected child.

Patients with primary Sjögren's syndrome are over 40 times more likely to develop haematological malignancy than patients of similar age and sex. These are usually B cell malignancies and should always be suspected in patients with swollen salivary glands.

Management

Lacrimal substitution should be given, by eye drops or liquid tears. These will help to reduce keratitis and eye ulceration. Treatment of oral symptoms is more difficult but saliva substitutes are available. Recent studies have sugested that pilocarpine can be useful in reducing symptoms, but this requires corroboration. Vaginal dryness can be treated with local lubricants and oestrogen creams. Systemic therapy includes hydroxychloroquine that can be beneficial if there is a significant skin rash and joint symptoms. Corticosteroids and immunosuppressants are only occasionally indicated in the presence of more serious manifestations. Appropriate therapy should be given for lymphomas if diagnosed.

MIXED CONNECTIVE TISSUE DISEASE

Mixed connective tissue disease (MCTD) is characterised by overlapping clinical features of SLE, progressive systemic sclerosis, polymyositis and an erosive arthritis akin to rheumatoid disease. It is characterised by a high titre of circulating auto-antibody against RNP. Clinical features include Raynaud's phenomenon, sausage swelling of the digits, skin changes resembling dermatomyositis or scleroderma, an inflammatory polyarthritis and often muscle weakness. Diffuse interstitial pulmonary fibrosis will infrequently occur but renal and CNS involvement is relatively rare.

Investigations in MCTD are those for the underlying disease, including ESR, muscle enzymes, rheumatoid factor and antibodies against RNP. Management is as for the component connective diseases and includes hydroxychloroquine, steroid therapy and immunosuppressive agents as required.

chapter 11

Systemic vasculitides

These uncommon diseases are characterised by an inflammatory cell infiltrate into the blood vessel wall. The vasculitis leads to blockage of vascular supply and necrosis of tissues distal to the obstruction. Vasculitis occurs secondary to a variety of inflammatory rheumatic diseases, such as SLE, systemic sclerosis, dermatomyositis, and Sjögren's syndrome. However the primary vasculitides are less common with a more serious form, such as Wegener's granulomatosis and microscopic polyarteritis being fatal if untreated. The aetiology of all these diseases remains unclear but hepatitis B

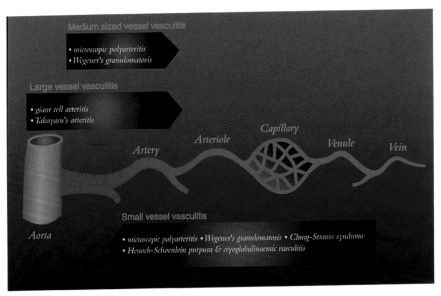

Figure 11.1 *Pattern for vascular involvement in vasculitides*

and C are commonly involved where these viruses are endemic. In any instance the key to the diagnosis is one widespread multi-system involvement, usually with severe constitutional symptoms with the size of blood vessel involvement dictating the symptoms and defining the disease character (Figure 11.1). In some vasculitides there are circulating antibodies directed against neutrophil cytoplasmic antigens (ANCA) (Figure 11.7 and 11.11). It is probably wise to refer all potential cases because of the difficulty in confirming the diagnosis.

In each case treatment is with high doses of steroids often with immunosuppression. Treatment with bisphosphonates is mandatory to reduce risks of osteoporosis.

LARGE VESSEL DISEASE

GIANT CELL ARTERITIS

(See also Chapter 12, polymyalgia rheumatica and giant cell arteritis.)

Clinical features

This is the commonest vasculitis in the United Kingdom. Most patients present with severe headache with scalp tenderness, anorexia, fatigue, weight loss, fever and general malaise.

The classical distribution involves the temporal and occipital vessels with tenderness over the inflamed vessel (Figure 11.2). However, the ophthalmic vessels can also be involved producing sudden blindness (amaurosis fugax) due to blockage of vascular supply (Figure 11.3). Vessels supplying the muscles for mastication can be obstructed causing jaw claudication, and transient ischaemic attacks may also occur from blockage of cranial vessels.

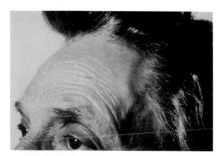

Figure 11.2 *Thickened temporal artery*

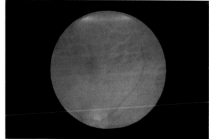

Figure 11.3 *Blocked ocular artery*

Investigation

Haematology The ESR is usually elevated well above 50mm.

Biochemistry The CRP mimics the ESR.

Histology Widespread cellular infiltration into temporal artery wall (Figure 11.4).

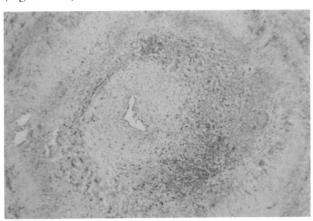

Figure 11.4 *Histology of temporal arteritis*

Differential diagnosis

Symptoms from giant cell arteritis can be mimicked by plaque embolisation from arteriosclerosis, systemic infections, and can occur as a result of a non-metastatic manifestation of underlying malignancy.

Treatment

Treatment is with systemic steroids, 50-60mg/day, started immediately if the clinical suspicion is high and the ESR confirms it. Gradual reduction in steroids over a three-month period, to between 10-20mg, guided by symptoms and the ESR is appropriate.

Maintenance therapy is required for at least one year and usually two. Rarely symptomatic relapses can occur, and if accompanied by a rising ESR, high dose steroids should be restarted and the use of steroids sparing immunosuppressive agents such as azathioprine or methotrexate should be considered.

The use of high dose steroid should be accompanied by appropriate treatment to prevent steroid-induced osteoporosis.

Epidemiology

The highest instance is in the elderly with a female:male ratio of 3:1. There are estimated to be 1.6–2.3 new cases per 100,000 population per annum.

TAKAYASU'S ARTERITIS

This large chronic inflammatory panarteritis classically affects the aorta and its major branches. It is characterised by constitutional symptoms, fevers, sweats, fatigue, weight loss, arthralgias and myalgias, together with anaemia. Because of the blood vessels involved, headaches, syncope, arm claudication and angina and classical symptoms and clinical examination reveals bruits, lack of pulses, hence its pseudonym pulseless disease. Systemic hypertension and aortic competence can occur. If severe myocardial infarction, transient ischaemic attack, cerebral vascular accident and upper limb ischaemia can occur.

Investigations

Haematology There is normochromic normocytic anaemia, leucocytosis, raised ESR.

Biochemistry The CRP mimics the ESR.

Radiology Chest x-ray will show widened aortic arch. Angiography will show stenosis in the aortic arch and its branches (Figure 11.5).

Histology Granulomas will appear with lymphocyte infiltration on biopsy.

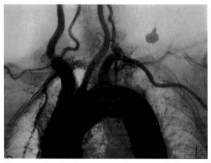

Figure 11.5 *Aortogram showing blockage of subclavian vessels in Takayasu's arteritis*

Treatment

Most patients respond to high dose oral prednisolone, 1-2mg/kg/day, but immunosuppression with cyclophosphamide, azathioprine or methotrexate may be required. Once vascular damage has occurred, reconstructive surgery may be necessary.

Epidemiology

Takayasu's arteritis affects primarily females aged under 40, with a high instance in the Far East and patients from Mexico. There is a probable genetic aetiology for this disease.

MEDIUM-SIZED VESSEL DISEASE

POLYARTERITIS NODOSUM

This vasculitis affects medium-sized blood vessels and may be related to patients with hepatitis-B, being more common in diseases where hepatitis-B infection is endemic.

Clinical features

Vague systemic illness, myalgias and mononeuritis multiplex, abdominal pains, arthritis, skin ulceration, purpuras, infarcts or gangrene. Hypertension and renal involvement imply a renal infarction. Testicular pain, leg and jaw claudication can occur as a result of vascular occlusion, and 30% of patients have lung involvement with chest pain and chest x-ray abnormalities.

Investigations

Haematology There is normochromic normocytic anaemia, raised ESR.

Biochemistry Abnormal renal function will appear with renal involvement or secondary to longstanding hypertension.

Microbiology Hepatitis B serology is often positive and hepatitis B antigen often present.

Immunology p-ANCA (Figure 11.7) is positive in 20% of cases, virtually always characterised as antibodies against the myeloperoxidase enzyme in neutrophils. The ANA and RhF are negative.

Radiology Chest x-ray may show isolated pulmonary infiltrate (Figure 11.6). Angiography will show multiple aneurysms in the coeliac access.

Pathology Biopsy of nerve, kidney or skin can show necrotising vasculitis.

Treatment

In the presence of hepatitis-B anti-viral therapy is appropriate, but immunosuppressive therapy with steroids and corticosteroids and

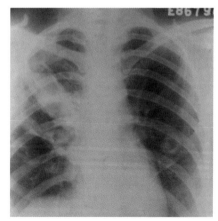

Figure 11.6 *Chest x-ray showing lung shadow*

cyclophosphamide has reduced the mortality from 100% down to around 20% over the past 20 years.

Epidemiology

The peak instance is between ages 40 to 50. Male:female ratio is 2:1. Incidence is three cases/million in most populations. It is therefore unlikely that there will be any patients in the average GP practice of 2,500.

KAWASAKI'S DISEASE

Clinical features

This is an extremely rare disease in Caucasians. Patients (usually children) present with an acute systemic vasculitis characteristically involving coronary arteries fever, acute non-purulent cervical lymphadenopathy, erythema of palms and soles with oedema and desquamation. Erythema of the lips, buccal mucosa and tongue occurs. Coronary aneuryms can develop with myocardial ischaemia with infarction, pericarditis, and pericardial diffusions.

Investigations

Haematology Leukocytosis, thrombocytosis and raised ESR are seen.

Biochemistry The CRP mimics ESR.

Immunology There are anti-neutrophil cytoplasmic antigens and anti-endothelial antibodies.

Radiology Coronary angiography demonstrates aneurysms.

Treatment

Treatment is usually with high dose intravenous gammaglobulin. Most children recover, with mortality of around 2%, and relapse is rare. Steroids should be avoided as this can worsen coronary disease.

Epidemiology

There is a very high incidence of Kawasaki's disease in Japan, with boys being affected three times more commonly than girls. It usually occurs under the age of five.

SMALL VESSEL DISEASE

MICROSCOPIC POLYARTERITIS

Clinical features

Patients with microscopic polyarteritis have predominantly renal and lung involvement. Systemic involvement, including peripheral nervous system and gastrointestinal tract, is less common than in classical polyarteritis nodosum. Renal impairment occurs in 90% of cases, but hypertension is only found in approximately 20% of patients.

Investigation

Haematology There is normochromic normocytic anaemia and raised ESR.

Biochemistry Renal function abnormality is seen. The CRP mimics ESR.

Immunology p-ANCA (myeloperoxidase) is positive in around 50% of cases (Figure 11.7).

Microscopy Casts appear in the urine.

Histology There is polyarteritis affecting glomerular capillaries, with no granulomas.

Treatment

Oral or intravenous prednisolone with cyclophosphamide are used to induce remission, dependent on results from blood white cell counts, which must be carefully monitored to avoid leukopaenia. Mesna is used to reduce the risks of intravenous boluses of cyclophosphamide inducing haemorrhagic cystitis and bladder cancer.

Following induction of remission, microscopic polyarteritis can be con-

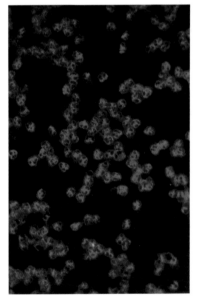

Figure 11.7 *p-ANCA*

trolled on a regime of a reducing dose of prednisolone, together with azathioprine. This therapy is usually continued for up to five years before withdrawal is considered because relapse rate is high.

Epidemiology

There is a slight male predominance and it is usually present in Caucasians but the incidence is only 3.6/million in the United Kingdom. It is a rare disease in the average general practice of 2,500.

WEGENER'S GRANULOMATOSIS

Clinical symptoms

Characteristically, systemic Wegener's granulomatosis presents with a triad of upper and lower respiratory tract granulomas with focal segmental necrotising glomerulonephritis. The pattern of clincial involvement is described in Figure 11.8. Common symptoms include nasal stuffiness and crusting (Figure 11.9),

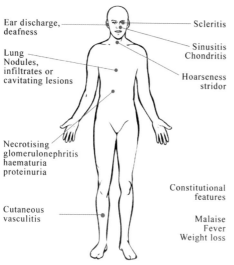

Ear discharge, deafness

Lung Nodules, infiltrates or cavitating lesions

Necrotising glomerulonephritis haematuria proteinuria

Cutaneous vasculitis

Scleritis

Sinusitis Chondritis

Hoarseness stridor

Constitutional features

Malaise Fever Weight loss

Figure 11.8 *Clinical features of Wegener's granulomatosis*

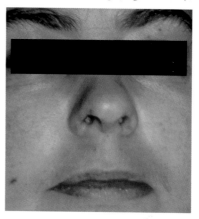

Figure 11.9 *Nasal crusting*
Figure 11.10 *Nasal deformity*

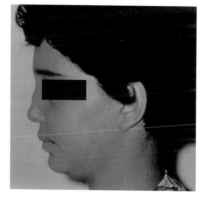

facial pain, epistaxis and middle ear symptoms with development of multi-system disease including renal impairment in 80% of cases. Laryngeal involvement, cough and haemoptysis are not uncommon due to the granulomas causing local obstruction or tissue damage that is most commonly seen in the nose (Figure 11.10). However, skin and joint involvement and neurological symptoms are less common than with polyarteritis nodosum. In the more limited forms of Wegener's granulomatosis symptoms are restricted to the upper and lower respiratory tract.

Investigations

Haematology There is normochromic normocytic anaemia, raised ESR,

Biochemistry Renal function abnormality is seen, with raised CRP.

Immunology There is cANCA (Figure 11.11) (characterised as proteinase 3) and complement consumption.

Histology There is necrotising vasculitis with granuloma, in ENT, lung or renal tissue (Figure 11.12).

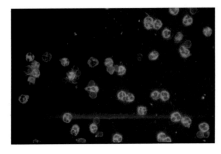

Figure 11.11 *c-ANCA*

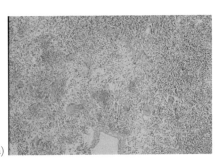

(a)

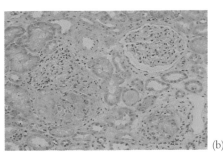

(b)

Figure 11.12 *Histology of Wegener's granulomatosis* (a) *shows infiltration of lung tissue with inflammatory cells and granulomata*, (b) *shows a focal segmental gomerulonephritis*

Treatment

Remission is induced with prednisolone and cyclophosphamide, dependent on results from full blood counts, which must be carefully monitored for leukopaenia. Mesna is used to reduce the risks of haemorrhagic cystitis and bladder cancer in patients receiving bolus chemotherapy with cyclophosphamide. Trimethoprim/sulfamethoxazole has been proven to be beneficial in limited forms of Wegener's granulomatosis, particularly those with upper respiratory tract diseases.

Epidemiology

Annual incidence of Wegener's granulomatosis is 8.5/million in the United Kingdom.

CHURG-STRAUSS SYNDROME

Clinical features

This vasculitis is characterised by long-standing history of allergic rhinitis with asthma, followed by an acute systemic illness with symptoms from pulmonary infiltrates (cough, breathlessness and haemorrhage), cutaneous skin rash (vasculitis) with neurological involvement (mononueritis multiplex).

Investigations

Haematology There is normochromic normocytic anaemia, raised ESR, eosinophilia.

Biochemistry Renal function abnormality is seen, with raised CRP.

Immunology There is complement consumption but ANCA, ANA RhF are negative.

Histology Vasculitis is seen with eosinophilic infiltration and giant cells.

Treatment

Remissions are induced using prednisolone and cyclophosphamide dependent on results from full blood counts, which must be carefully monitored for leukopaenia. Mesna is used to reduce the risks of haemorrhagic cystitis and bladder cancer in patients receiving bolus chemotherapy with cyclophosphamide. Reduction in prednisolone dose is gradual, but patients may need to remain on low doses with azathioprine to prevent relapse.

Epidemiology

The overall incidence of Churg-Strauss syndrome is 3.3/million in the United Kingdom. Five-year survival was initially reported at approximately 62%, in response to steroids alone. This has increased with the use of immunosuppressive agents.

LEUCOCYTOCLASTIC VASCULITIS

This blood vessel inflammation affects small and medium blood vessels in the skin and occurs secondary to drug reaction, serum sickness, infections, malignant tumours, usually in the absence of any internal organ involvement.

Investigations include elevation of acute phase response, complement consumption, and unless these are secondary to underlying disease, such as SLE and Sjögren's syndrome, auto-antibodies are usually negative. Skin biopsy shows vasculitis with dying white cells with pycnotic nuclei.

HENOCH-SCHONLEIN PURPURA

This classical, purpuric rash occurs usually but not exclusively in children less than five years old. The rash (Figure 11.13) is usually located over the lower limb, often on the posterior aspect of the buttocks and thighs and may be associated with arthritis, gastrointestinal involvement with gastrointestinal bleeding and rarely glomerulonephritis. Systemic involvement with fever malaise and weight loss is around 50% in children. This is usually a self-limiting disease.

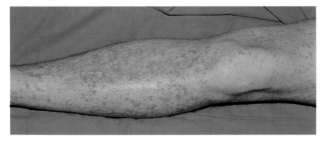

Figure 11.13
Microscopic vasculitis

Complement consumption is not uncommonly associated with an elevated acute phase response. When occuring in adults the renal involvement is said to be as high as in 75% of cases, which is associated with IgA antibodies present in the kidney biopsy.

Steroids are reserved for systemic involvement.

CRYOGLOBULINAEMIA

Cryoglobulins are circulating immunoglobulins that precipitate in the cold. Features are associated with cryoglobulinaemia include purpura, urticaria, cutaneous ulceration, arthralgias, rarely glomerulonephritis, peripheral neuropathy, lymphadenopathy and liver dysfunction (often associated with an underlying hepatitis-C infection).

Cryoglobulins can be classified into the monoclonal forms associated with myeloma, lymphoma or Waldenstrom's macroglobulinaemia or polyclonal, which are usually associated with underlying hepatitis-B or hepatitis-C infection. These can be differentiated by protein electrophoresis.

Treatment with steroids, immunosupressants, plasmaphoresis or high dose globulins have all been tried, but the prognosis tends to be poor.

BEHÇET'S SYNDROME

This is a rare vasculitis in the Western European population, although a genetic association with HLA-B5 has been reported. Major criteria include oral ulceration, genital ulceration, uveitis and skin lesion associated with pathergy (pustules at the sites of venepuncture). Other minor criteria include inflammatory arthritis at the large joints, intestinal ulceration, epididimyitis, thrombophlebitis and meningoencephalitis.

Investigations show an elevated acute phase response but essentially they are limited to excluding other forms of systemic vasculitis. Management includes symptomatic treatment. Colchicine can be used for oral ulceration. Corticosteroids are often required but recently the use of thalidomide is becoming increasingly popular to help control symptoms.

chapter 12

Polymyalgia rheumatica and giant cell arteritis

(*See also Chapter 11, systemic vasculitides.*)

Polymyalgia rheumatica can be a difficult condition to diagnose in primary care and yet can be one of the most satisfying to treat.

CLINICAL FEATURES

Polymyalgia rheumatica is a clinical syndrome comprising a number of different features including:

- stiffness and pain in shoulder and pelvic girdles;
- associated systemic features of debility, weight loss, tiredness and low grade fever;
- raised ESR.

The diagnosis of polymyalgia rheumatica can be supported by a dramatic response to cortico-steroids. Stiffness is often the main feature and there may be some tenderness of the affected muscles. The joints themselves are not usually affected.

Polymyalgia rheumatica tends to occur in patients aged over 50 with a peak incidence at around 70 and it occurs twice as often in women as in men. It affects around 20 to 70 persons in every 100,000 aged over 50 years.

Polymyalgia rheumatica may present suddenly with a dramatic onset of stiffness and pain sometimes coming on almost overnight or in other cases with a much more insidious onset with less in the way of stiffness and pain and more in the way of systemic features. If there is a relatively sudden onset of symptoms with a raised ESR and a dramatic response to steroid therapy the diagnosis can usually be made with confidence. In patients with an insidious onset and with several systemic features the diagnosis can be difficult and a wide range of differential diagnoses may have to be considered.

Giant cell arteritis occurs in around 10 to 20 persons per 100,000 of the population with a mean age of onset at 70 and an incidence which rises with increasing age. As with polymyalgia rheumatica, females are affected three times as often as males. Giant cell arteritis is a condition which has an overlap with polymyalgia rheumatica. Symptoms of arteritis may develop during the course of polymyalgia rheumatica and in some patients with polymyalgia rheumatica, biopsy may show the characteristic pathological changes of arteritis. It is thought that these two conditions represent opposite ends of the spectrum of the same disease with polymyalgia rheumatica at the milder end and giant cell arteritis at the more severe end. The pathological changes in giant cell arteritis show a giant cell infiltrate with thickening of the intima of the artery and restriction of the lumen.

In giant cell arteritis, the patient usually presents with headache which is often severe. This headache usually has a sudden onset and affects the temporal regions although it may also be occipital or generalised. Scalp tenderness is often present together with jaw claudication. Visual symptoms, including visual loss, diplopia and ptosis are especially important. Examination may reveal tender, thickened temporal arteries (Figure 12.1) which may show reduced or absent pulsation. The ESR is usually raised. The danger of giant cell arteritis is that it may lead to visual loss and blindness and indeed, permanent loss of sight occurs in around 20% of cases. For this reason giant cell arteritis must be treated urgently with an adequate dose of corticosteroid. If giant cell arteritis is suspected most primary care physicians would refer immediately to a specialist who would usually perform a temporal artery biopsy (Figure 12.2). If there is likely to be any delay in referral it is safer to start treatment with steroids prior

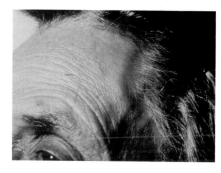

Figure 12.1 *Thickened temporal artery*

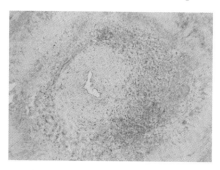

Figure 12.2 *Histology section of affected artery*

to being seen in secondary care to avoid visual complications. Around one third of patients with giant cell arteritis will have a negative biopsy. This does not mean that the diagnosis is wrong, as it may be difficult to obtain affected material in what may be a very localised area of pathological change.

Although the chances of obtaining a positive biopsy decrease rapidly with steroid therapy, treatment should not be delayed for the sake of obtaining a biopsy as the patient would then be at risk of permanent visual problems and possibly blindness.

DIAGNOSIS

Although the ESR is usually significantly raised in both polymyalgia rheumatica and giant cell arteritis there are documented cases where the ESR is normal or only a little raised. These cases may cause diagnostic difficulties and while the diagnosis on clinical grounds may well be correct it is obviously important to consider other conditions. Similarly, in patients with suspected polymyalgia rheumatica who present with systemic features, other causes of illness should be excluded. Rheumatoid arthritis can have a polymyalgic presentation and may be very difficult to distinguish from polymyalgia rheumatica. If there are peripheral joint signs such as synovitis the diagnosis is most likely to be that of rheumatoid arthritis as joint synovitis is relatively rare in polymyalgia rheumatica. If a patient diagnosed as polymyalgia rheumatica fails to respond to steroids or if you are not able to reduce the dose of steroid from the initial dose without exacerbation of symptoms, a diagnosis of rheumatoid arthritis is much more likely.

DIFFERENTIAL DIAGNOSIS OF POLYMYALGIA RHEUMATICA

- multiple myeloma
- other malignancy
- rheumatoid arthritis
- connective tissue disease
- osteoarthritis
- myopathy
- myositis
- hypothyroidism
- osteomalacia
- fibromyalgia
- shoulder problems (e.g. capsulitis or tears of the rotator cuff)

INVESTIGATIONS

It is worth remembering that no specific test is diagnostic for polymyalgia rheumatica and that the diagnosis remains based on clinical findings and on exclusion of other conditions as appropriate.

ESR (or PV) is the single most usual investigation and, if raised, tends to support the diagnosis of polymyalgia rheumatica. C-reactive protein is usually also raised. Patients with polymyalgia rheumatica often have a normocytic anaemia and a raised alkaline phosphatase. If this is the case and the patient has some systemic symptoms malignancy should be considered and a chest x-ray performed. There is an association of hypothyroidism with polymyalgia rheumatica and thyroid function tests should also be taken to exclude this.

Some doctors would suggest that all patients should have protein electrophoresis or immunoglobulins assessed to exclude multiple myeloma. Again if there is any doubt about the diagnosis it is worth checking rheumatoid factor although, if positive, this is not necessarily diagnostic for rheumatoid arthritis. If disease of muscles, such as polymyositis, is suspected it is worth checking muscle enzymes, e.g. creatine kinase.

Investigations for suspected polymyalgia rheumatica

- ESR;
- FBC;
- LFT;
- thyroid function tests;
- protein electrophoresis;
- rheumatoid factor.

Investigations for suspected giant cell arteritis

- ESR;
- FBC;
- LFT;
- temporal artery biopsy.

MANAGEMENT

Straightforward cases of polymyalgia rheumatica can be treated satisfactorily within primary care. If there are no contraindications, patients should be started on 15mg prednisolone per day. This should bring rapid relief of symptoms within a few days.

If this does not happen, a re-think of the diagnosis is needed.

The dose of prednisolone should then be reduced to 12.5mg/day after four weeks and then to 10mg per day after a further four weeks and then titrated down slowly according to symptoms rather than to ESR. The dose can be reduced by 1mg per day down to 5mg daily over six to 12 months. Normally, once 5mg daily is reached, the dose should be reduced more slowly, aiming to have the patient steroid free by around two years, although some patients may require a small dose of steroids for three to four years.

Any relapse of symptoms should be treated by increasing the dose again and then titrating down more slowly. If it is not possible to reduce the steroid dose down without exacerbating the symptoms or if the patient suffers several relapses it is important to consider another diagnosis especially rheumatoid arthritis.

In giant cell arteritis the initial steroid dose is much higher, usually starting at around 50-60mg daily for one week and reducing to 40mg daily for a further two weeks. After this and depending on response, it may be possible to reduce the daily dose by 10mg each week down to 20mg daily and then by 2.5mg each week down to 10mg daily. Then the dose can be gradually reduced as in polymyalgia rheumatica. Any exacerbation of symptoms will mean that a temporary increase in dosage is required followed by a slower reduction of dose. Again the aim of treatment is to wean the patient off prednisolone over two to three years.

Dosage regimes vary according to the individual doctor and the individual response of the patient. Most physicians however are agreed on the starting doses of prednisolone as 10-20mg per day for polymyalgia rheumatica and 40-60mg per day for giant cell arteritis.

Some patients with polymyalgia rheumatica can be treated with NSAIDs alone but response is often poor and corticosteroid therapy is certainly the treatment of choice. As corticosteroid therapy is weaned off some patients may benefit from a small dose of NSAID at this stage to alleviate some of the minor muscle pain that sometimes ensues.

Initial dosage regime

This should be 10-20mg daily for polymyalgia rheumatica, 40-60mg daily for giant cell arteritis.

Complications of therapy

It is important to assess the patients for their risk of osteoporosis in view of the steroid intake. If possible a DEXA scan should be obtained and treatment initiated if appropriate. High dose of steroids can also cause gastric irritation and some gastro-protection may be required.

Relapses

Relapses are fairly common in polymyalgia rheumatica and should be diagnosed on clinical rather than laboratory grounds. They may occur as a response to too rapid a decrease in the dose of corticosteroid. Various studies report relapse rates of between 30–60 % and it is thought that the chances of relapse are higher in the first six to 12 months of treatment.

PROGNOSIS

The long-term prognosis of polymyalgia rheumatica is good and many patients can discontinue their steroid treatment in around two year's time with no long-term sequelae. Some patients, however, will need longer treatment and may require to stay on a small dose of steroids for several years. The necessity for prolonged therapy seems to be greater with increased age at diagnosis, in females, and in those with a higher initial ESR.

Patients should be warned about the possibility of the development or return of visual symptoms and advised to report any such symptoms immediately.

REFERRAL

For polymyalgia rheumatica, consideration should be given to referring patients:

- who have a poor response to steroids;
- in whom it is difficult to reduce the steroid dose;
- in whom the diagnosis is unclear;
- who have repeated relapses.

For giant cell arteritis, all patients should be referred to a specialist immediately but steroid treatment should not be delayed where there may be delay in the patient being seen. It is safer to treat first to avoid visual loss.

chapter 13

Fibromyalgia

Fibromyalgia is a syndrome rather than an actual disease. It occurs commonly, particularly in women and is often very difficult to manage. No specific pathology has been demonstrated in patients with fibromyalgia and for many years patients with this syndrome have been thought to have a psychosomatic basis for their symptoms or indeed to be imagining them. As characteristic features of fibromyalgia have been recognised making it easier to make a diagnosis, there has been an increase in interest in the condition with a subsequent improvement in management.

CLINICAL FEATURES

These include:

- musculo-skeletal pain, often widespread and affecting back and neck;
- may be associated with generalised mild morning stiffness;
- pain may be made worse by stress;
- patient may complain of 'pain all over';
- pain is rarely alleviated by analgesics or NSAIDs;
- fatigue is often severe and after only minimal exertion;
- there is usually sleep disturbance giving non-restorative sleep;
- psychological distress;
- multiple tender sites which are hyperalgesic;
- subjective feeling of swelling of digits;
- headache and abdominal pain;
- irritable bowel and irritable bladder symptoms;
- poor memory and difficulty concentrating.

AETIOLOGY

The cause of fibromyalgia is not known. There seems to be an overlap with chronic fatigue syndrome. At various times viral infections and musculo-skeletal trauma have been thought to be associated with the development of the condition. Patients with fibromyalgia often show marked psychological distress and it has been mooted that this may be the cause of the development of the syndrome. It is difficult to ascertain whether the psychiatric illness gives rise to the development of fibromyalgia or whether it develops as a response to the distress felt by the sufferer.

DIAGNOSIS

There are no specific laboratory tests for fibromyalgia, which is basically a clinical diagnosis. Obviously many conditions may have some of the clinical features associated with fibromyalgia and it is important to exclude any other important diagnoses.

DIFFERENTIAL DIAGNOSIS OF FIBROMYALGIA

- inflammatory arthritis;
- systemic lupus;
- hypothyroidism;
- malignancy;
- polymyalgia rheumatica;
- inflammatory myopathy;
- hyperparathyroidism.

Laboratory tests may be useful to exclude some of the above conditions. These might include:

- FBC;
- ESR;
- thyroid function tests;
- ANA;
- serum calcium;
- creatine kinase.

Patients with fibromyalgia often do not look ill and it is frequently difficult to correlate their physical signs with their apparent disability.

It is important to make a positive diagnosis as this is the first step in management and means that the patient can hopefully move on to some understanding of the condition and to taking some positive steps to deal with it. An early diagnosis may also prevent the patient from attending multiple outpatient appointments and undergoing many negative investigations.

A positive diagnosis should include:

- 11 or more hyperalgesic sites;
- demonstration of some non-tender control sites;
- normal clinical examination.

Table 13.1 Tender sites in fibromyalgia

Tender sites/trigger points:

- low cervical spine
- low lumbar spine
- suboccipital muscle at base of skull
- trapezius at mid-point
- supraspinatus
- skin roll tenderness over mid trapezius

- lateral epicondyle
- greater trochanter
- medial fat pad of knee
- gluteus medius
- second costochondral junction

The first three sites mentioned above occur in the midline whereas the others occur bilaterally.

Everyone has some sites on the body which are uncomfortable when pressed or rolled firmly under a finger. In a patient with fibromyalgia light pressure in these areas produces an exaggerated response of extreme pain and wincing. Relevant sites are shown in Table 13.1 and Figure 13.1. In order to make a

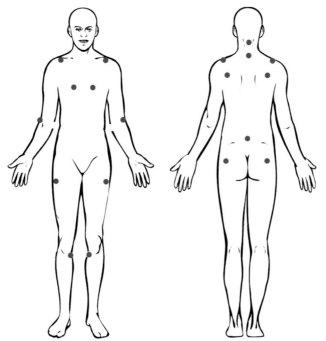

Figure 13.1 *Diagram of tender sites / trigger points*

diagnosis there should not be a response of this nature at other 'non-tender' sites such as the forehead. If the patient does respond in an exaggerated way at the 'non-tender' sites the diagnosis is not fibromyalgia but a possible psychiatric problem or a complete fabrication of symptoms.

MANAGEMENT

This condition is one that produces a negative attitude in many doctors. Some doctors do not really believe that the condition exists and management started on that basis is almost doomed to fail. It is important first of all to show sympathy for the patient and convey that you believe that they are experiencing real pain and disability. It is also important to reassure the patient that they do not have a serious disease in terms of pathology. The fact that you can give a diagnosis and a name to their condition can be helpful in itself. Education as to the nature of the condition both to the patient and to their family is very valuable. The patient's drug regime should be reviewed and any unnecessary or ineffective medication should be stopped. Any other associated conditions such as irritable bowel are worth treating and it is sometimes a good idea to try amitriptyline at night in a low dose to improve the sleep pattern. Patients should be encouraged to try a gradual aerobic exercise plan. This is often resisted by the patients who believe that they are not fit enough to try this and that exercise will exacerbate their condition. It is true that there probably will be an increase in muscle pain at the start of an exercise programme but this is a normal response of muscles to unaccustomed exercise and patients should be encouraged to continue with the advice that they will not do themselves any damage. Some patients will benefit from referral for psychological support and may be encouraged to learn some coping strategies. Teaching cognitive and behavioural techniques can produce considerable benefit for some patients and help to reduce their pain and distress.

It is important to try to encourage patients to take some control themselves in terms of their own condition and to dissuade them from becoming dependent on doctors and on continually requesting new referrals to different specialists and seeking new medications to help their pain symptoms.

PROGNOSIS

The prognosis in fibromyalgia is not very good. Many patients are unable to hold down a job and the condition often has an adverse effect on all aspects of their life. Some patients however manage to control some of their symptoms and while not actually cured of the problem they succeed in coming to terms with it and so improving their quality of life.

REFERRAL

- Patients should be discouraged from repeated referral to secondary care.
- Referral to clinical psychologist may be appropriate.
- Complementary medicine may be helpful.

chapter 14

Musculo-skeletal problems in children

General practitioners are often consulted by parents who bring along a child with a musculo-skeletal problem. This may range from an abnormality of gait to a complaint of pain from the child. Many of these problems are simple and require only reassurance but as in so many areas of medicine, it is important to be aware of red flags and other potential problems. The child may be too young to give any sort of history and clinical signs may be confusing. Most GPs see only a very few children with serious musculo-skeletal pathology and so it is difficult to build expertise in dealing with these uncommon and potentially difficult problems. If there is any doubt the child should be referred for an expert opinion.

Categories of diseases causing musculo-skeletal problems in children include:

- inflammatory: juvenile chronic arthritis, connective tissue disease, inflammatory bowel disease etc.;
- mechanical;
- infection;
- trauma including non-accidental injury;
- metabolic, endocrine and dietary;
- haematological;
- tumours;
- hypermobility syndrome;
- idiopathic pain syndromes, e.g. growing pains (nocturnal idiopathic musculo-skeletal pain syndrome), reflex sympathetic dystrophy, fibromyalgia.

INFLAMMATORY CONDITIONS

Juvenile chronic arthritis

Juvenile chronic arthritis (JCA) is a relatively rare condition occurring in 1 in a 1,000 children, although many of these patients will have only mild disease. Most GPs see very few new presentations and diagnosis can be difficult in the early stages. Symptoms are variable and young children often cannot express what they feel wrong.

The presenting signs The child may present with a variety of features, specific such as limping, or non-specific such as fever, loss of appetite, irritability or rash. Joint swelling or synovitis may be difficult to discern in young children and pain is not necessarily a main feature.

There are a number of other conditions which can cause similar preceding symptoms in children. Infective conditions, such as septic arthritis and osteomyelitis should be considered as a differential diagnosis. In an ill child, with an acute joint swelling, it is essential to exclude infection. If there is any doubt, the child should be admitted to hospital immediately for further investigation.

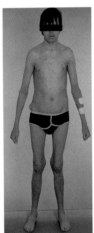

The management of juvenile chronic arthritis should be undertaken by specialist paediatric rheumatologists with input from a specialist multi-disciplinary team although it is nevertheless important that the child's general practitioner is aware of the management options so that he or she can support the family through what is often a very difficult time(Figure 14.1).

Figure 14.1 *Child with juvenile chronic arthritis*

There are three main classifications of JCA:

Systemic onset (10% of total) This occurs most commonly between ages one to five. It usually remits in six months. 50% of patients have recurrent attacks, 25% go on to develop severe chronic polyarthritis. Presenting signs and symptoms include arthralgia, polyarthritis, failure to thrive, fever, rash, lymphadenopathy, hepatosplenomegaly, and retardation of growth.

Polyarticular (30% of total) In this group, four or more joints are involved. One-third of this group are seronegative and of these 10-15% will go on to develop severe arthritis. Two-thirds are seropositive. Here the onset is usually over eight years of age and 50% will go on to develop erosive arthritis. Clinically the picture is similar to that of adult rheumatoid arthritis.

Pauciarticular (60% of total) In this group fewer than four joints are involved and 70% will have complete resolution of the condition. There are two main groups, young girls (40% of total) and older boys (20% of total). In the young female group HLA-DR5 is commonly found and half of these children are found to be ANF positive. This is regarded as a marker for chronic iritis. In the older male group 75% are HLA–B27 positive and there is often a family history of a seronegative disorder. In this group lower limb joints are commonly affected and sacroiliitis may occur.

Management of JCA

Analgesics and NSAIDs are usually required especially when synovitis is present. Intra–articular steroids can be very useful but this should always be a hospital procedure.

Sometimes DMARDs are initiated and occasionally shared care for monitoring is requested but mostly this is undertaken in a hospital environment. Much of the management of JCA centres around physical therapy using exercise regimes, hydrotherapy, and splinting. Education and advice on joint protection, aids and appliances and environmental adjustments are also extremely important. JCA can cause immense problems for both the affected child and for the family and both may require psychological support. School age children may also suffer much disruption of their education and educational support is very important.

Connective tissue disease

Conditions such as juvenile dermatomyositis and SLE are relatively rare in children but could be considered as a differential diagnosis for musculoskeletal problems. Henoch-Schonlein purpura is a vasculitis which presents as an arthritis of the larger joints with abdominal pain and a purpuric rash usually over the legs and buttocks. A few children with this condition develop nephritis and this may lead to chronic renal failure.

Other inflammatory joint disease

Psoriasis and inflammatory bowel disease can cause an inflammatory joint disease in children.

Reactive arthritis

This can occur quite commonly in children following an episode of infection such as:

- gastrointestinal infection e.g. salmonella, shigella, campylobacter;
- viral infection e.g. rubella, coxsackie B, herpes, parvovirus, hepatitis B;
- lyme disease;
- post streptococcal.

MECHANICAL PROBLEMS

Mechanical abnormalities include:

- congenital dislocation of the hip;
- flat feet;
- in-toe/out-toe gait;
- valgus or varus abnormalities at the knee.

Congenital dislocation of the hip

If congenital dislocation of the hip (CDH) (Figure 14.2) is not picked up early, this may cause limping, unequal leg length and late standing or walking with a waddling gait. It is important to recognise CDH to avoid problems in later life, such as arthritis at the hip.

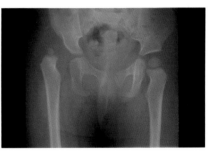

Figure 14.2 *X-ray of congenital dislocation of the right hip*

Risk factors for CDH:

- family history;
- breech delivery;
- presence of other congenital deformities;
- low birth weight or foetal growth retardation;
- cerebral palsy;
- racial background e.g. CDH common in North American Indians but rare in Africa.

Babies should be examined at birth, at six weeks, and at eight months and usually Ortolani's test is used. It is important not to over-manipulate the hips of a small baby as this can occasionally cause damage.

If a clink is heard or felt, the child should be referred immediately for an expert opinion. Management consists of placing the hips in a reduced abducted position such as shown in the older child in Figure 14.3. For minor problems in infants, double nappies are sometimes sufficient. For major problems, including those in older children, plaster or splints may be required for up to 15 months.

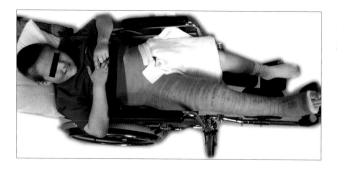

Figure 14.3 *Hip in reduced abduction position*

Legg-Perthes disease

Legg–Perthes (Perthes) disease (idiopathic osteonecrosis of the femoral head)tends to occur in three to 12 year olds, although it is more common in males aged five to eight. It is bilateral in around 10% and affects boys three to five times as often as girls. The affected child is very often small for its age and has a delayed skeletal age compared to the chronological age. Around 10% have a family history of the problem.

Symptoms are sudden onset of limping often with very little pain. If there is pain it is often referred to the knee and this can cause difficulties in diagnosis. Sometimes the child will present with refusal to weight bear, limping or fever. The differential diagnoses include irritable hip and septic arthritis. X-ray shows classical features of flattening of the femoral head (Figure 14.4). Only around 60% of affected children will require specific treatment while the rest will need only symptomatic treatment. Management includes analgesics and NSAIDs if required, crutches and short term night-time traction and reduction in activities. In more severe cases braces or surgery are required to produce 'containment' of the femoral head.

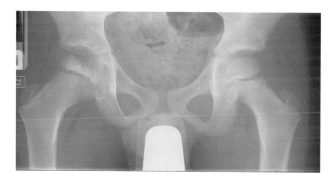

Figure 14.4 *X-ray of right hip with Legg-Perthes disease*

INFECTION

Septic arthritis

This is uncommon but potentially very serious and should be considered as a differential diagnosis in all children who have joint pain and swelling together with fever.

Osteomyelitis

Children below the age of one year with this condition usually present with a septicaemia and joint swelling and tenderness. Older children are not willing to weight bear on the affected limb and usually show signs of localised infection such as tenderness, swelling and warmth. If diagnosed and treated early the prognosis is good with little in the way of long term complications.

Irritable hip

This is a benign, self-limiting condition which can be confused with sepsis. Irritable hip is most common in males, aged four to seven, and there is often a preceding upper respiratory tract infection in the previous two weeks. The illness may last from a few days to a few weeks. The child is non-febrile and often limping and on examination there may be some guarding on movement of the hip. If there is any doubt about the diagnosis the child should be referred to hospital.

TRAUMA

In most significant injuries the child is taken straight to hospital. Sometimes, however, the injury did not appear to be serious at the time and the child presents at the surgery on the following day with pain and stiffness and is brought to exclude a fracture.

Non-accidental injury (NAI) to children is unfortunately not an uncommon occurrence. GPs have to have a high index of suspicion for NAI to babies and children and if there is any doubt as to the cause of an injury the child should be sent to hospital immediately.

METABOLIC, ENDOCRINE AND DIETARY CONDITIONS

Conditions such as rickets, insulin dependent diabetes mellitus, scurvy and hyper- and hypothyroidism can give rise to chronic diffuse musculo-skeletal pain in children. Adequate treatment of the underlying condition usually solves the problem.

HAEMOGLOBINOPATHIES

This group of conditions includes such diseases as sickle cell disease and b-thalassaemia. The underlying problem is vaso-occlusion and this can lead to dactylitis and osteonecrosis. Dactylitis can occur in young children and presents with acute painful swelling of hands and feet. The condition usually improves in a week or so and generally causes no long term problems. Children may also develop osteonecrosis of the femoral head. This causes pain on weight-bearing and symptoms tend to last over several weeks. Although there may be flattening of the femoral head children often retain good function compared with adults with the same condition where there is often a progressive deterioration of joint function.

TUMOURS

Malignant

Haematological malignancies such as lymphoma and leukaemia can give joint and muscle pain in children, while tumours of bone and cartilage, fortunately rare, can give localised pain in joints.

Benign

The most common benign bone tumour of childhood is an osteoid-osteoma (Figure 14.5). They present between the ages of five and 30 and often occur in the proximal half of the femur. They frequently give night pain and on examination there is sometimes some atrophy of the muscles of the thigh and unequal leg length. The main differential diagnosis of an osteoid-osteoma is growing pains (see below). Management is usually surgical removal.

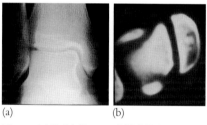

(a)   (b)

Figure 14.5 (a) *X-ray and* (b) *MRI scan showing osteoid osteoma of right fibula*

HYPERMOBILITY

Hypermobility often first becomes evident in childhood. In this condition the ligaments around the joint are lax and the individual may then suffer problems due to over-extension of the joint and trauma to the tissues. Mildly hypermobile individuals may have no symptoms while others, more severely affected, may suffer from a range of joint and back pain.

NON-ARTHRITIC LOCOMOTOR DISORDERS

Idiopathic musculo-skeletal pain syndromes

Idiopathic pain syndromes tend to be stress-related. They are more common in pre-adolescent females. There are various background factors, such as pushy parents, dysfunctional families, over achievement in academia or sport and sexual abuse. Management includes education, physical therapy, psychological support, and possibly analgesics, NSAIDs and amitriptyline, although these should be discontinued as soon as possible.

Growing pains (nocturnal idiopathic musculo-skeletal pain syndrome)

Growing pains tend to occur in five to 13 year olds. The pains are worse at night and often waken the child from sleep. They usually occur in the lower limbs but may occur elsewhere around the body. The attacks last for 15 to 30 minutes and may be relieved by massaging the limb. They are sometimes precipitated by increased exercise on the previous day but characteristically there are no symptoms on the following day. If the child has symptoms on waking, the diagnosis is unlikely to be growing pains and another pathology should be sought. With growing pains there is usually nothing to find on examination and the management consists of reassurance and analgesics. Growing pains may be stress related and are sometimes associated with abdominal pain or headache.

Reflex sympathetic dystrophy

This condition is due to abnormal autonomic function. The patient presents with pain and tenderness in a limb which is often pale and mottled in colour with a decreased skin temperature and possibly some soft tissue swelling. Although uncommon it occurs more frequently in pre-adolescent girls than in other paediatric age groups.

Fibromyalgia

In this condition there is usually considerable stiffness and pain at several sites, with multiple painful trigger points and an abnormal sleep pattern with complaints of waking feeling tired due to non-restorative sleep. There may be an association with hypermobility.

Part 3

COMMON MUSCULO-SKELETAL PROBLEMS

chapter 15

Back pain

Back pain is a very common reason for a patient to seek a consultation in primary care. Many of these presentations are for acute and short term conditions but a significant number become a chronic problem, often with no demonstrable pathology and with little response to common management techniques.

Most patients with back pain can be treated within primary care but there are some important signs and symptoms, which should alert you to a possible 'red flag' requiring further investigation or referral.

PREVALENCE

On any specific day around 25% of all adults will have some degree of low back pain and 75% of all adults will have an episode of low back pain during their lifetime. Back pain is more common in females and the prevalence rises with increasing age up to around age 55.

Musculo-skeletal disorders are the commonest cause of chronic disability and more than 50% of this is due to back pain. There are a huge number of days lost from work because of back pain and this appears to be increasing. Back pain itself does not seem to be more prevalent in industrialised countries but the concept of disability due to back pain certainly is. This appears to result from a view in developed countries that low back pain is an illness rather than part of normal life.

AETIOLOGY OF SIMPLE MECHANICAL LOW BACK PAIN

In most cases the actual cause of back pain in pathological terms is not known. There is sometimes a relationship to injury but this is not always obvious.

Risk factors for the development of low back pain:

- increased height;
- poor muscle strength;

- poor physical fitness;
- unequal leg length;
- heavy physical work or work with much twisting, lifting or bending;
- work involving sitting and driving for long periods;
- smoking.

The rationale for the influence of smoking is not clear but it is thought possibly to be due to increased pressure due to repeated coughing.

PROGNOSIS OF LOW BACK PAIN

Seemingly similar presentations of low back pain in different people can result in different outcomes with the acute problem resolving in some but becoming chronic in others. These different outcomes are thought to be due partly to the influence of psycho-social factors.

30% of cases of low back pain will resolve within two days and 90% within six weeks. After this time period the chances of a full recovery with a return to work decrease considerably.

The longer a patient is absent from work the less the chances of a return to employment. After one year of absence from work only 30% are likely to return and after two years only 10 %. It is therefore important that those involved in primary care do everything possible to prevent back pain developing into a chronic problem and provide active intervention and encourage a return to work as soon as possible.

DIAGNOSIS OF BACK PAIN

There are three main questions to be answered from history and examination:

- Is the pain coming from a musculo–skeletal problem in the spine or is it arising from another organ? Pain in the back may arise from lungs, kidneys, stomach or pelvic organs.
- Is the pain mechanical or otherwise?
- Are there any neurological features?

Taking a history in back pain

History should include:

- age;
- site of pain;
- type of pain;
- aggravating features;
- alleviating features;
- radiation;
- history of previous episodes;
- obvious precipitating events;
- past medical history;
- present general health;
- interference with work or leisure activities;
- any sleep disturbance;
- any medication taken;
- any physical therapy used.

'Red flags'

Red flags are points in the history or examination of a patient with back pain which would alert the doctor to a potentially serious condition.
Another diagnosis should be considered if:

- the patient is younger than 20;
- the patient is older than 55 with no past history of relapsing backache;
- the pain affects the thoracic region;
- the patient is generally unwell with weight loss and/or other systemic symptoms;
- there is marked early morning stiffness;
- the pain is constant and unremitting;
- past medical history includes carcinoma or osteoporosis;
- medication includes present or past corticosteroids;
- there is a significant history of injury;
- there are widespread neurological symptoms.

Other potential diagnoses

Malignancy

This may be primary especially myeloma, or secondary due to metastatic spread especially from carcinoma of breast, prostate, lung and kidney. Patients are often ill with severe unremitting pain and weight loss.

Infection

Spinal abscess is uncommon but may occur in the elderly and may be due to tuberculosis.

Inflammatory disease

The most common inflammatory disease affecting the spine is ankylosing spondylitis although psoriatic arthritis and enteropathic arthritis can also show spinal involvement. Suspect an inflammatory disorder if the onset of the pain is gradual with early morning stiffness. There may also be peripheral joint involvement and symptoms relating to other body systems e.g. iritis, psoriasis, or colitis.

Osteoporotic fracture

Contrary to many patients perceptions, osteoporosis is not painful unless there has been a fracture of the bone. This may be only a minor fracture within the bone but can, nevertheless, be extremely painful. A past history of relevant risk factors for osteoporosis would suggest the possibility of this diagnosis. These might include present or past corticosteroid use, previous low trauma fracture, oestrogen lack, thyrotoxicosis, alcohol abuse, smoking, low body weight, malabsorption syndromes, anorexia.

Neurological disorder

If there are widespread neurological signs and symptoms affecting more than one nerve root this is not radicular pain and the possibility of a neurological disorder should be considered. Cauda equina syndrome is a condition where patients present with pain associated with difficulties with micturition, faecal incontinence, numbness around the perineum and anus (so-called 'saddle anaesthesia') and motor weakness in the legs. More than one nerve root is affected .

Paget's disease

Paget's disease of bone may give back pain.

CLASSIFICATION OF BACK PAIN

Having decided that the pain is coming from the spine it is then important to classify it further. 90% of all back pain is due to simple mechanical backache, while 9% has nerve root pain and 1% is due to a spinal problem.

Examination

A good history (see above) should provide with some indications on how to examine the patient and which investigations might be undertaken.

If there are any features suggesting a serious spinal pathology then a full examination and investigation is essential. Most patients, however, will have simple backache and with an extremely common and usually benign condition it would not be possible to examine each of these patients fully at every surgery visit within the time constraints that exist.

It is important, however, to perform an initial screening examination, especially on patients presenting with back pain for the first time, to exclude any obvious problems.

Assess the patient's general demeanour. Does he look ill? Can he sit comfortably and stand up straight? Does he appear to be obviously in pain? Does he limp? Watch him as he lies up on the examination couch and assess which movements seem to provoke pain.

Ask the patient to strip to undergarments and look at the spine. Is there a normal lumbar lordosis? Check forward flexion, extension, side flexion and rotation. Assess lumbar flexion by asking the patient to bend forwards and mark the lumbar spine in two places with two fingers. Ask the patient to stand up and look at his or her fingertips. Flexion of the lumbar spine should mean that the two marks come closer to each other. If there is an inflammatory condition such as ankylosing spondylitis then the two marks will stay apart at the same distance indicating a fixed lumbar spine with poor or nonexistent flexion. Ask the patient to lie on his back on the examination couch. Check straight leg raising (SLR). In the young normal patient this is normally 90° and pain free. SLR is limited by pain in nerve root problems and raising the affected leg reproduces the pain. SLR may also be limited by poor musculature in the posterior thigh. If SLR is positive raise the leg to the limit of the patient's pain and then flex the foot. This should produce an exacerbation of the patient's pain by stressing the nerve root

With the patient on the couch look for any signs of muscle wasting although this would be an unusual finding in an acute backache as it generally is a later development and suggests a lower motor neurone lesion. Assess reflexes, power and sensation as appropriate. The knee jerk relates to L3/4 while the ankle jerk relates to S1. When checking reflexes remember to check both sides. Table 15.1 shows the effects of lumbo sacral root lesions. Figure 15.1 shows the distribution of the dermatomes. Low back pain in itself can give rise to generalised tenderness over the spine. Specific areas of moderate to severe tenderness, however, might suggest another spinal pathology such as an osteoporotic fracture.

If any features are present suggesting other pathology then a full physical and neurological examination is essential with other investigations as appropriate.

Table 15.1 Lumbo-sacral root lesions

root	sensory loss	motor weakness	affected reflex
L4	calf and ankle medial aspect	extension of knee inversion of foot	knee
L5	medial foot and great toe	dorsiflexion of foot and great toe	—
S1	lateral side of foot and sole	plantar flexion of foot	ankle

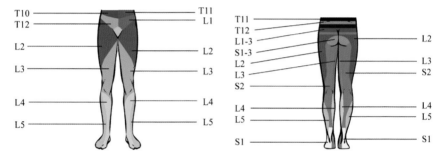

Figure 15.1 *Distribution of the dermatomes of the lower limb*

SIMPLE BACK PAIN

Simple back pain is most common in the 20 to 55 age group. If the patient is younger, or older with no history of previous relapsing backache, it is important to consider an alternative diagnosis.

Characteristics of simple backache:

- usually aged 20 to 55;
- usually involves the lumbar region;
- usually made worse by activity and relieved by rest although some patients find their pain is helped by walking and made worse by sitting;
- the patient is generally well in himself;
- simple backache can be associated with referred pain felt across the buttocks and possibly spreading to the thighs and even down to the knee.

Management of simple back pain

Simple back pain is generally managed in primary care. Management initially consists of patient education and prescription of simple analgesia. Analgesia should be taken regularly to facilitate movement and to keep the patient as active as possible. If simple analgesics are insufficient to control the pain then compound analgesics and/or NSAIDs may be used. Bed rest should be avoided but if necessary should be limited to a maximum of three days. If possible patients should remain at work or if time off work is necessary they should be encouraged to return as soon as possible. If pain persists after a week or two more active intervention is required with referral for physical therapy and/or manipulation. If the patient is still off work and in pain after six weeks it is important:

- to reassess the diagnosis;
- to consider any psychosocial factors.

RISK FACTORS FOR THE DEVELOPMENT OF CHRONIC BACK PAIN

These include:

- previous history of low back pain;
- previous loss of work due to low back pain;
- leg pain;
- decreased SLR;
- nerve root involvement;
- poor physical condition;
- smoking;
- depression;
- psychological distress;
- personal problems with relationships, alcohol, money;
- poor job satisfaction;
- poor self esteem;
- any medico–legal situation pending, e.g. compensation.

If the patient is not back at work within three months this could be considered a failure of primary care management and the patient should be referred for further treatment. Where the patient is referred depends to a large extent on local facilities. Physiotherapy is often the initial referral and should be considered for any patient who has not already received some physical therapy. Some areas have a back pain rehabilitation service, which is generally multidisciplinary. It may also be appropriate to refer for help with pain management perhaps to a pain clinic where again there may be a multidisciplinary team including clinical psychologists and anaesthetists.

In some areas the back pain service is run by rheumatologists and in other areas by orthopaedic surgeons.

RADICULAR PAIN (NERVE ROOT PAIN)

Radicular pain or nerve root pain may be caused by a prolapsed intervertebral disc, spinal stenosis or scarring. Radicular pain gives unilateral leg pain usually radiating to the foot or toes, and associated with paraesthesiae and numbness. The patient usually shows signs of nerve irritation. SLR is decreased and reproduces the leg pain. Neurological signs relating to power, sensation and reflexes are confined to one single nerve root. Radicular pain is often sharp and severe and can be very distressing for the patient to the extent that associated back pain is often ignored. Around 50% of patients with nerve root pain recover from an acute attack within six weeks.

Initial management is similar to that of low back pain although the patient may require a short spell of bed rest and stronger analgesia. If the patient has severe or progressive motor weakness then referral to an orthopaedic surgeon is advised. Again, if the pain does not improve after six weeks referral should be considered.

INVESTIGATIONS

There are no specific investigations for low back pain. If another condition is suspected then appropriate investigations should be performed including blood tests and imaging as required. Patients often request a back x-ray. This should be discouraged. Plain x-rays of the lumbar spine are of little value and give 120 times as much radiation as a chest x-ray so should not be performed as a routine. It may however be appropriate to x-ray in some circumstances, such as thoracic pain or if another pathology is suspected. Remember though that x-rays may be normal even in the presence of serious spinal pathology and referral should not be delayed on this basis. Other imaging techniques such as MRI and CT scans may be more appropriate investigations for nerve root problems and serious spinal pathology.

SUMMARY OF MECHANICAL BACK PROBLEMS

- Simple backache.
- Prolapsed intervertebral disc: gives radicular pain, neurological signs and decreased SLR.
- Facet joint pain: unilateral, worse on exercise and on rotation and side flexion.
- Spondylolisthesis: slippage of one vertebra on another. May be due to a congenital problem or degenerative changes. Instability of lumbar spine may give neurological involvement.
- Spinal stenosis, due to a decrease in space within the vertebral canal. May be congenital but usually acquired as a space-occupying lesion in a narrow canal due to a disc prolapse or to degenerative changes. Spinal stenosis gives leg pain which is worse on walking, relieved by rest and by bending forwards and discomfort in legs at night giving cramps and restless legs. Differential diagnosis is with vascular claudication where peripheral pulses are absent or diminished. Management is conservative unless symptoms are very severe, when surgery is indicated
- Sacroiliac strain: pain is generally felt in a localised area in the upper medial buttock. Pain may be due to a strain of the strong ligaments, which bind the sacrum to the ilium. Many specialists, however, are sceptical of the existence of this condition.
- Coccydynia: usually caused by injury. If there is no response to analgesia, infiltration with steroid and local anaesthetic can be very effective. Very occasionally surgery is indicated to remove the coccyx.

MANAGEMENT BY THE MULTIDISCIPLINARY TEAM

Many back pain teams comprise members of different specialities but the actual mix of expertise may vary from area to area. Treatments may include analgesics, NSAIDs, antidepressants and occasionally muscle relaxants. Local anaesthetic and steroid injections may be used. These injections may include epidural and caudal injections and also injections into trigger points. Various physical modalities in use include TENS, electrotherapies, acupuncture and lumbar supports. Some pain clinics have a clinical psychologist who can help patients to come to terms with their pain and to develop some coping skills and self-efficacy.

Surgery to the spine

Few patients require surgery to the spine and indeed this is best avoided if possible. Indications for surgery include:

- acute spinal cord damage;
- acute cauda equina syndrome;
- widespread neurological disorder;
- nerve root problem not resolving with conservative management.

Referral

Reasons for referral are as follows:

- in mechanical back pain if no better after two to three weeks refer for physical therapy;
- if still in pain and not back at work in six weeks, consider psycho–social assessment;
- if still in pain at three months, refer to local back pain service, including pain clinic for rehabilitation and pain control;
- patients with 'red flags' may need referral to the appropriate specialist in secondary care;
- refer to surgeons if relevant indication (see above);
- refer to rheumatologist if inflammatory disease suspected.

chapter 16

Neck pain

Although figures suggest that neck pain causes only about one-tenth of the disability caused by back pain, neck pain is nevertheless a common presentation in primary care and often becomes a recurrent problem. As in low back pain, although most neck pain is due to a mechanical problem it is important to exclude 'red flags' and systemic causes.

DIFFERENTIAL DIAGNOSIS OF NECK PAIN

Consider:

- mechanical problem;
- malignancy: myeloma, metastatic disease;
- inflammatory: rheumatoid arthritis, ankylosing spondylitis, polymyalgia rheumatica;
- infection;
- other causes: fibromyalgia, shoulder problems.

TAKING A HISTORY FOR 'RED FLAGS' IN NECK PAIN

Ask about:

- any history of injury;
- systemic symptoms;
- unremitting and progressive pain;
- history of rheumatoid arthritis;
- past history of malignancy;
- severe restriction of range of movement of cervical spine;
- corticosteroid therapy;
- history of osteoporosis;
- any leg symptoms;
- multiple neurological changes.

In simple mechanical neck pain there are often predisposing factors in the past history such as a history of whiplash injury, heavy or unaccustomed lifting or carrying or different and unaccustomed household tasks. Carrying heavy shopping, painting a ceiling or hanging heavy curtains may all precipitate acute neck pain.

When asking about neck pain it is important to ascertain:

- site and character of the pain;
- any radiation;
- duration of pain;
- any relieving or aggravating features;
- any past history of neck pain and its outcome;
- any symptoms of vertigo;
- any treatments already tried.

In patients with vertigo associated with neck pain it is important to exclude a vertebral or basilar artery cause. If these arteries are compressed when the patient turns his head, this produces symptoms of vertigo. If this is the case manipulation as a treatment for neck pain is contraindicated.

EXAMINATION OF PATIENTS WITH NECK PAIN

Look at the patient's general appearance, in particular the posture. Many people nowadays spend long periods of time in front of a computer screen, which may not be positioned correctly. This can lead to poor posture and muscle spasm across the back of the neck and the shoulders and give rise to neck pain.

Feel the neck for muscle spasm and any localised tenderness. Assess the range of movement of the neck both active and passive and check flexion, extension, and lateral flexion and rotation to both sides. It is helpful to assess shoulder movements at the same time and this can be done quickly by using a GALS system.

If there is any arm pain or any neurological symptoms in arms or legs a neurological examination should be carried out. Arm pain may be due to a trapped nerve or to nerve irritation.

The vast majority of neck pain with root signs affects C5-C8 with C7 involvement being the most common (Table 16.1). Figure 16.1 shows the distribution of the dermatomes in the upper limbs.

Table 16.1 Cervical root lesions

root	reflex depressed	motor weakness	sensory loss
C5	biceps	shoulder abduction	outer arm to base of thumb
	supinator	elbow flexion	
C6	biceps	elbow flexion	anterior lateral arms, thumb and index finger
	supinator	wrist extension	
C7	triceps	elbow extension	posterior arm, middle three fingers
C8	none	finger flexion ulnar deviation wrist thumb adduction and extension	ring and little fingers

Flexion of the cervical spine may exacerbate symptoms of cord compression while extension of the cervical spine may cause an exacerbation of root symptoms. Compression of the cord gives upper motor neurone signs in arms and legs.

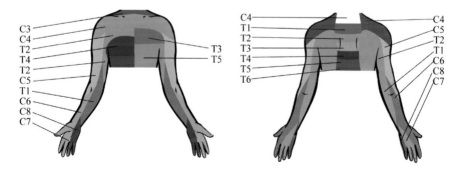

Figure 16.1 *Distribution of the dermatomes of the upper limb*

RHEUMATOID ARTHRITIS

Long standing rheumatoid arthritis affects the cervical spine in around 25% of patients. Joint laxity may give instability and atlanto-axial subluxation (Figure 16.2). This can cause cord compression. Surgical treatment may be appropriate in some cases while a rigid collar is also useful. At risk patients should take care to avoid whiplash injuries and should wear a collar while travelling in a moving vehicle.

WHIPLASH INJURIES

These injuries occur when a moving vehicle comes to a sudden standstill causing a jerk to the neck of any passengers. Such injuries are most usual when a car is hit from behind but may also occur with side or front collisions. The commonest injury seems to be due to forced extension of the cervical spine. The patholog-

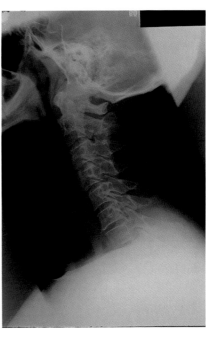

Figure 16.2 *X-ray of cervical spine in rheumatoid arthritis, showing subluxation at the atlanto-axial joint*

ical changes are thought to be due to stretching or tearing of ligaments and muscles. X-rays are often performed especially in hospital A&E Departments but rarely show any relevant abnormalities. Most patients aged over 40 will have some degenerative changes on x-ray in any case and are usually asymptomatic. Management of whiplash injury is similar to that of other neck pain with the emphasis on analgesia and early mobilisation. The greater use of head restraints has helped to reduce this problem but it remains a common cause of neck pain and is often slow to resolve. In around 10% of those affected, symptoms are still present after six months. There is frequently a psychological aspect to whiplash injuries that fail to resolve. This may be due to post-traumatic stress following the accident or may be associated with insurance or compensation problems.

INVESTIGATIONS OF NECK PAIN

X-rays are rarely helpful unless severe trauma is suspected. MRI scans can be useful for imaging cervical disc problems such as prolapse. If a non-mechanical cause is suspected for neck pain then other relevant investigations should be carried out.

MANAGEMENT OF NECK PAIN

As in low back pain, modern management of neck pain includes analgesia with the emphasis on early mobilisation. Cervical collars are often provided particularly after a whiplash injury but should only be used during activities which exacerbate pain and use should if possible be restricted to a few weeks. Some patients with recurrent neck pain find that intermittent use of a collar during exacerbations of pain is an effective intervention. If abnormal posture is a predisposing factor advice should be given to correct this. Mobilisation, perhaps with manipulation, is an effective therapy and referral to a physiotherapist or to a chiropractor or osteopath is usually helpful. Traction is sometimes used for more resistant problems.

REFERRAL

Reasons for referral are as follows:
- if simple neck pain is not settling within a few weeks refer for physical therapy for mobilisation;
- if there are neurological problems, refer to surgeons;
- if suspected inflammatory disease, refer to rheumatologist;
- if suspected malignancy, infection or other 'red flag' refer to appropriate specialist.

chapter 17

Monoarthritis

A patient with a single swollen joint can present a considerable diagnostic challenge. Sometimes the diagnosis is obvious from the patient's history and examination but often the situation is less clear cut.

The first most important rule is to exclude potentially very serious conditions or 'red flags'. Septic arthritis is the most important of these conditions.

SEPTIC ARTHRITIS

Risk factors for septic arthritis include:

- recent intra-articular injection;
- diabetes;
- rheumatoid arthritis;
- HIV infection;
- systemic infection;
- immuno-compromised patients;
- malignancy;
- pre-existing joint prosthesis;
- drug addiction;
- sexual promiscuity (gonococcus).

Remember that both corticosteroid therapy and NSAID therapy can mask signs and symptoms of infection.

If septic arthritis is not rapidly and adequately treated it can produce rapid joint destruction and may be fatal.

Patients with a monoarthritis due to sepsis usually have constitutional symptoms such as fever. The affected joint is red, hot, swollen and shiny, tender to touch and very painful to move (Figure 17.1). If sepsis is suspected the patient should immediately be referred to hospital where the joint should be aspirated and synovial fluid obtained, if possible before starting intravenous antibiotic therapy. Gram staining of the synovial fluid helps to select the most appropriate antibiotic initially though of course this may need to be

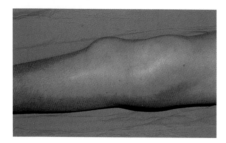

Figure 17.1 *Septic arthritis of the right knee*

changed following culture. Unless there are unusual circumstances antibiotics should not be started without obtaining a synovial fluid sample as this may result in partial treatment of the condition which may then continue to lead to subclinical joint destruction. Antibiotic therapy often has to be continued for four to six weeks and the joint may require repeated aspiration. Once the joint has settled clinically, gentle physiotherapy can be started to regain function and movement.

DIFFERENTIAL DIAGNOSES

The main differential diagnoses of septic arthritis are:

- gout and pseudogout;
- trauma.

Gout

Gout (see Chapter 7) can also produce a red, hot shiny joint which will also be exquisitely tender to touch and very painful to move. The patient while in considerable discomfort does not however have the constitutional signs of sepsis such as fever. If gout is suspected it is always advisable to aspirate the joint and look at the fluid through a polarising microscope. A history of recurrent episodes of acute arthritis would support a diagnosis of gout and while monoarticular gout may occur in any joint it is most commonly seen in the first MTP joint, although 30% will get their first attack in hand, knee, other joints of the foot or the shoulder.

Pseudogout

Pseudogout (see Chapter 7) is caused by shedding of pyrophosphate crystals into the joint from articular cartilage. This condition shows up as chondro-calcinosis on x-ray. The clinical picture is of an acute arthropathy but is usually not as acute or as painful as gout and most commonly affects knee, wrist or shoulder. Diagnosis again is by aspiration of synovial fluid and microscopy.

Trauma

Trauma sufficient to produce a monoarthritis is usually obvious from the history, although sometimes a definite history of injury is difficult to obtain especially in the elderly. Sometimes a relatively minor injury can give rise to a haemarthrosis, which can be diagnosed by aspiration of blood stained synovial fluid. Haemophilia and pseudogout may also cause haemarthrosis.

Other causes of monoarthritis include:

■ tick–borne disease e.g. lyme disease;
■ viral related disease e.g. rubella. This may occur after an attack of rubella or after vaccination and is more common in adults.
■ inflammatory
■ non–inflammatory

Inflammatory joint disease may also present as a monoarthritis although this is much less common than the typical polyarthritis. Rheumatoid arthritis, psoriatic arthritis, Reiters disease and ankylosing spondylitis may all present in this way. Joints may be inflamed, swollen and tender but are not usually red and hot as in sepsis.

Non–inflammatory conditions may also give a monoarthritis. The most usual cause is osteoarthritis. Commonly there is a history of pain and stiffness in the joint over some time and the joint may show the chronic changes of osteoarthritis such as bony swelling, crepitus and possibly 'squaring'. The joint looks a normal colour and usually feels cool, although there may be warmth during an inflammatory flare. An effusion may be present and this may have been aggravated by mild trauma or increased activity. During an inflammatory flare in an osteoarthritis joint there is often increased pain, swelling and tenderness, but unless there is sepsis present the joint is not 'hot' and red.

chapter 18

Pain all over

'Doctor, I've got pain all over' is a frequently heard symptom in GPs' consulting rooms. It is often difficult to diagnose at one visit and may require several clinical assessments and perhaps some laboratory investigations before being able to reach a diagnosis. With conditions such as fibromyalgia, generalised osteoarthritis and post-viral syndrome laboratory investigations are often performed to exclude rather than to confirm certain conditions and to reassure the patient. Often all investigations are normal and it is then sensible to check for psychosocial factors and to assess the impact of stress in the patient's background. Many conditions presenting with 'pain all over' are associated with malaise and non-restorative sleep.

It is of course very important to assess fully these patients, as sometimes pain all over can be the initial presenting symptom of a potentially very serious condition, such as malignancy, which may manifest itself as time goes on.

Depression and anxiety in themselves may lead to a complaint of 'pain all over'. The reverse also occurs where a chronic painful arthritic condition such as generalised osteoarthritis, inflammatory arthritis (Figure 18.1) or SLE leads on to the subsequent development of depression and anxiety because of chronic pain and decreased functional ability. In these conditions, clinical examination and laboratory tests will generally be helpful in establishing the diagnosis.

Common conditions giving 'pain all over' seen in primary care are:

- fibromyalgia;
- post-viral syndrome;
- generalised osteoarthritis;
- inflammatory arthritis;
- polymyalgia rheumatica;
- depression and anxiety;
- multiple regional pain syndrome.

Less commonly seen conditions include:

- SLE;
- hypothyroidism;
- malignancy, especially multiple myeloma;
- Paget's disease;
- osteomalacia;
- myositis.

With the complaint of pain all over, it is obviously important to take a full history and perform a full clinical examination.

If a systemic disease is suspected, the appropriate investigations should be performed and obviously once a diagnosis is confirmed appropriate management should be instigated.

Depression and anxiety may respond to counselling and explanation, although antidepressant medication may be required by some patients. Post-viral syndrome has no specific treatment although some sufferers do become depressed (whether this is cause or effect is often difficult to ascertain) and again antidepressants may be needed.

Fibromyalgia should be managed as described in Chapter 13 and multiple regional pain syndromes should be treated as each individual separate lesion.

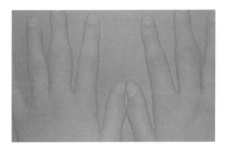

Figure 18.1 *Acute polyarthritis in rheumatoid arthritis*

Shoulder problems

Shoulder pain is a common presenting problem especially in the elderly, and can cause considerable disability. Some estimates suggest that 25% of all elderly patients suffer from shoulder pain. This can be very restrictive in maintaining independence and may also cause disturbed sleep, as the affected shoulder is often painful to lie on. Many of these shoulder problems can be managed successfully in primary care but before any management plan can be put in place it is important to diagnose accurately the cause of the pain and to tailor the therapy accordingly.

Conditions causing pain around the shoulder are:

- rotator cuff tendinitis;
- rotator cuff tear;
- subacromial bursitis;
- adhesive capsulitis (frozen shoulder);
- bicipital tendinitis;
- rupture of long head of biceps;
- acromio-clavicular lesions;
- reflex sympathetic dystrophy;
- osteoarthritis of the shoulder joint;
- rheumatoid arthritis;
- polymyalgia rheumatica;
- fibromyalgia;
- referred pain from cervical spine;
- referred pain from heart, lungs or diaphragm;
- bone pain from metastatic spread.

The history of the problem is obviously important. There may be a history of trauma or unaccustomed activity at home or at work. It is also important to know where the pain is, if it radiates and any exacerbating or relieving factors. Pain in the upper part of the arm generally comes from the shoulder whereas pain over the top of the shoulder often comes from the cervical spine (Figure 19.1).

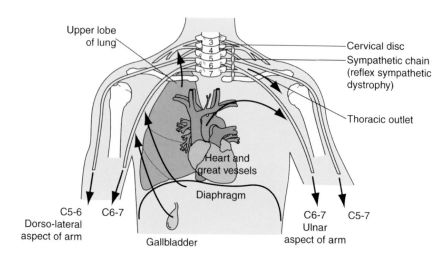

Upper lobe
of lung

Cervical disc
Sympathetic chain
(reflex sympathetic
dystrophy)

Thoracic outlet

Heart and
great vessels

Diaphragm

C5-6   C6-7
Dorso-lateral
aspect of arm

Gallbladder

C6-7   C5-7
Ulnar
aspect of arm

Figure 19.1 *Distribution of pain arising from the neck and from the shoulder*

In order to diagnose a shoulder problem in the short time available within a primary care consultation, it is important to devise a quick and effective routine for shoulder examination.

Ask the patient to undress to the waist. Check active movements of both shoulders assessing abduction, internal and external rotation, flexion/abduction, and the scarf test (Figure 19.5). If there is any restriction of active movement, reassess by passively repeating the movement. Note any pain or restriction of movement. If any of the above movements produce pain, then by checking resisted active movement it may be possible to identify the individual muscle involved. In practical management terms this is usually not necessary but it can be satisfying to achieve. If shoulder movements are normal remember to assess the cervical spine. If the range of movements at the cervical spine is also normal consider another cause of pain such as referred pain from another organ, bony pain from a metastatic tumour or pain from polymyalgia rheumatica or fibromyalgia.

COMMON SOFT TISSUE PROBLEMS AROUND THE SHOULDER
Rotator cuff tendinitis
The rotator cuff of the shoulder comprises four muscles and their tendons: supraspinatus, infraspinatus, teres minor and sub-scapularis. The rotator cuff

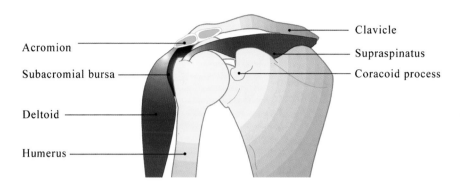

Acromion

Subacromial bursa

Deltoid

Humerus

Clavicle

Supraspinatus

Coracoid process

Figure 19.2 *Bony and soft tissue structures around the shoulder*

is subject to many strains and stresses and problems relating to the rotator cuff form the largest group of conditions causing shoulder pain. In patients of all ages tendinitis is common and in older patients this may be accompanied by degenerative changes which may lead to partial or complete rupture of the cuff.

Affected patients usually complain of pain in the upper arm, which often disturbs their sleep. There is usually a painful arc (Figure 19.3) on abduction of the arm, active movement is often limited and resisted movement produces pain and localised tenderness at the insertion of the cuff. Management includes rest with avoidance of any precipitating activities, analgesics, and anti-inflammatory drugs if necessary. Steroid injection into the subacromial space is often an effective intervention. A painful shoulder quickly becomes stiff, particularly in the elderly, and it may be very difficult to recover full mobility within the joint. Steroid injection can facilitate early mobilisation and can reduce the need for drug therapy. This is an important consideration, again especially in the elderly who often have concurrent illnesses and are taking concomitant medication.

Tears can occur in the rotator cuff and are usually the result of acute trauma in younger

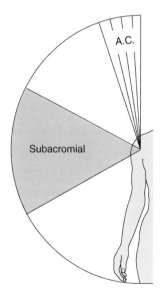

Figure 19.3 *Painful arc*

patients or relatively minor trauma to an already degenerate cuff in older patients. If there is a complete tear, the 'drop' sign is positive. To demonstrate this, place the patient's arm at 90° of abduction. If a tear is present the patient is unable to hold the arm in this position and the arm will drop to the side. Such tears are usually managed conservatively but if there is continuing pain and disability surgical repair may be required especially in younger patients. This can sometimes be performed arthroscopically but may require open reduction.

Subacromial bursitis

This condition may arise on its own or may be associated with a rotator cuff tendinitis. The subacromial bursa lies between the head of the acromion and the supraspinatus tendon. If bursitis is present the patient will demonstrate pain on movement of the shoulder with signs of a painful arc and tenderness over the shoulder area. The most effective treatment is steroid injection into the subacromial bursa. If local anaesthetic is used in the injection and the injection is correctly sited, the patient should be able to abduct the arm with no pain following injection, although the pain may recur when the local anaesthetic wears off. Sometimes the injection needs to be repeated after four weeks or longer for maximum effectiveness.

Adhesive capsulitis (frozen shoulder)

This condition is associated with gross restriction of movement especially external rotation. It is most common in females aged 50 to 60. It may arise for no obvious reason although many cases are associated with conditions which give rise to immobilisation of the shoulder such as rotator cuff lesions or strokes. Capsulitis is also more common in diabetic patients.

There appear to be three stages of frozen shoulder. First, the development of capsulitis with pain and loss of mobility; secondly, the development of adhesions giving the 'frozen' and immobile stage, and thirdly, the stage of gradual recovery. The natural history of frozen shoulder is resolution within two to three years and patients can be reassured that they will eventually recover. Management includes analgesics and anti-inflammatory drugs, if required, physiotherapy and mobilisation. Steroid injection into the gleno-humeral space can be effective especially if given before the 'frozen' stage develops. Very occasionally manipulation under general anaesthetic is required.

Bicipital tendinitis

This is inflammation of the tendon of the biceps muscle. In this condition the patient complains of pain around the front of the shoulder and there is tenderness over the tendon as it lies in the bicipital groove which is on the antero-lateral aspect of the upper arm. Resisted flexion of the elbow is painful. Conservative treatment with rest, physiotherapy and analgesics or anti-inflammatory drug therapy usually relieves the problem but resistant cases may require a steroid injection into the tendon sheath. If this is the case care must be taken to ensure that the injection is into the sheath and not the tendon as there is a danger of tendon rupture.

Rupture of the long head of biceps

In this case the history is usually of a sharp pain occurring on lifting. On examination there may be some bruising present and on flexing the elbow against resistance a bulge appears in the upper arm, the so-called 'Popeye' sign (Figure 19.4)

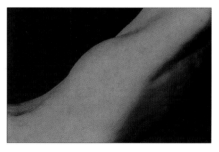

In younger patients surgical repair is the treatment of choice while in older patients conservative manage-ment is usual with initial rest

Figure 19.4 *Ruptured long head of biceps*

followed by early mobilisation. The short tendon of the biceps muscle continues to work and provides a degree of function.

Acromioclavicular joint lesions

Osteoarthritis is a common occur-rence in this joint. Some cases are thought to be due to previous injury especially from sports such as rugby or throwing sports. There is usually tenderness over the joint with some swelling. Raising the arm above 90° of abduction gives pain as does moving the arm across the front of the chest to the top of the opposite shoulder: the so-called 'scarf' test (Figure 19.5). If conservative manage-

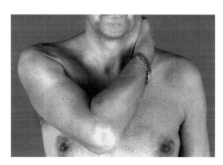

Figure 19.5 *'Scarf' test stressing the right acromioclavicular joint*

ment with analgesics, anti-inflammatories and rest fails to solve the problem most cases will respond to a steroid injection into the joint. The joint space is very small and only 0.2–0.4 ml volume is required. This can be a most effective intervention and often results in a very grateful patient.

Reflex sympathetic dystrophy (shoulder-hand syndrome) (RSD)

In this condition of unknown aetiology, the patient complains of pain in the shoulder and the arm and hand although most clinical signs are found in the hand. RSD is associated with restriction of movement and tends to occur following such conditions as a stroke, myocardial infarct, fracture or herpes zoster. RSD tends to have a gradual onset a few weeks after the precipitating event. Although RSD may give shoulder pain it is usually associated with signs and symptoms in the hand (Figure 19.6). Symptoms are of a burning pain in the arm and hand with swelling, redness and increased sweating of the hand followed by a change of appearance to a white colour with shiny skin. At this stage there may be some muscle atrophy and x-rays may show some

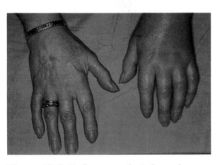

Figure 19.6 *Reflex sympathetic dystrophy (RSD) of the left hand*

patchy osteoporosis. Management of this condition is difficult and if not successful can result in a totally useless hand. These patients should therefore be referred for specialist input, including physiotherapy and treatment with calcitonin or bisphosphonates. If this is not effective sympathetic block may be useful. Acupuncture, TENS, splinting and antidepressants may also have a place in treatment.

Other conditions causing shoulder pain

These include:

- osteoarthritis: many older patients will have some changes of osteoarthritis of their shoulders on x-ray but these are generally asymptomatic. More severe symptoms can be associated with shoulder osteoarthritis although this is relatively uncommon and may be related to previous trauma. Management is as for osteoarthritis in other areas;
- rheumatoid arthritis often affects the shoulder joints and can cause considerable disability but frequently responds to steroid injection;
- polymyalgia rheumatica causes pain and stiffness in the shoulders but is always bilateral;
- referred pain from other structures;
- nerve entrapment syndromes;
- brachial neuritis: in this condition of unknown aetiology pain and restric-

tion of movement leads on to muscle wasting around the shoulder. Management is conservative and the condition generally resolves in around two to three years.

'RED FLAGS' FOR SHOULDER PAIN

Consider:

- trauma: fracture, dislocation;
- infection, especially in patients with rheumatoid arthritis;
- capsulitis and frozen shoulder: check urine for sugar;
- referred pain from other structures.

chapter 20

Elbow problems

Common soft tissue problems around the elbow are:

- lateral epicondylitis (tennis elbow);
- medial epicondylitis(golfer's elbow);
- olecranon bursitis.

LATERAL EPICONDYLITIS

This condition causes pain and tenderness over the lateral condyle of the elbow at the site of the common extensor tendon's attachment to the bone (Figure 20.1).

Inflammation in an area such as this where a tendon is attached to a bone is known as an enthesopathy. Lateral epicondylitis is usually unilateral and the patient complains of pain around the lateral aspect of the elbow, sometimes radiating into the forearm or upper arm. On examination there

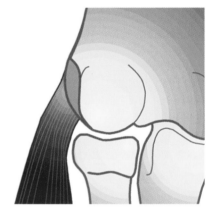

Figure 20.1 *Lateral epicondylitis*

is tenderness over the area where the tendon inserts into the lateral epicondyle. Resisted extension of the wrist reproduces the pain. Pain may range from mild and intermittent to fairly severe causing sleep disturbance and difficulty lifting. Management is rest and identifying and removing any precipitating factors. Oral and topical NSAIDs may have some benefit but the most effective treatment is steroid injection into the point of maximal tenderness. This can be a painful procedure and the patient should be warned that the pain may last for a day or two. Patients should also be advised of the risk of skin atrophy with this relatively superficial injection. A short acting steroid is best used in this situation to try to prevent this occurrence. The injection may need to be repeated if there is no resolution of the symptoms although this should not be repeated more than three times and in each case only after an interval of four weeks. Other treatments include physiotherapy and ultrasound, and in very severe and chronic cases, manipulation under general anaesthetic.

MEDIAL EPICONDYLITIS

This is similar to lateral epicondylitis except that it occurs at the common flexor origin on the medial aspect of the elbow (Figure 20.2). Again there is localised tenderness and resisted flexion of the wrist reproduces the pain. Management is as for lateral epicondylitis. When injecting for medial epicondylitis it is important to avoid injecting into the ulnar nerve which normally runs just behind the medial epicondyle.

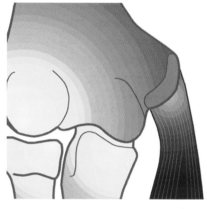
Figure 20.2 *Medial epicondylitis*

If patients complain of bilateral pain in the elbows this is unlikely to be due to epicondylitis and another diagnosis should be considered such as rheumatoid arthritis or osteoarthritis.

OLECRANON BURSITIS

In this condition patients present with a soft and sometimes tender swelling over the tip of the elbow (Figure 20.3). This can be caused by repeated trauma, such as continual leaning on the elbows, or may be associated with an inflammatory condition such as rheumatoid arthritis or with a crystal arthropathy. Management consists of avoiding any precipitating factor and

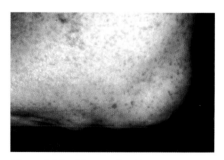
Figure 20.3 *Olecranon bursitis*

resting the area. Any underlying condition should be identified and treated as appropriate. Aspiration is sometimes useful especially for diagnostic purposes to exclude crystals or infection. Often the bursa fills up again after aspiration. Recurrent problems are sometimes treated with aspiration followed by the injection of a small dose of steroid.

chapter 21

Wrist and hand problems

Wrist and hand problems are common presenting problems in primary care. Some of these problems are due to underlying generalised or systemic conditions such as inflammatory arthritis, osteoarthritis or gout and these conditions together with referred or radicular pain from the neck or shoulder, trauma and reflex sympathetic dystrophy (RSD) should be considered as differential diagnoses for a soft tissue problem in this region.

COMMON SOFT TISSUE PROBLEMS AROUND THE WRIST AND HAND

These are:

- carpal tunnel syndrome;
- trigger finger;
- mallet finger;
- De Quervain's tenosynovitis;
- Dupuytren's contracture;
- ganglion.

OTHER DIFFERENTIAL DIAGNOSES

Consider:

- inflammatory arthritis;
- osteoarthritis;
- gout;
- trauma;
- reflex sympathetic dystrophy;
- neck or shoulder conditions.

CARPAL TUNNEL SYNDROME

This is caused by entrapment of the median nerve as it passes under the flexor retinaculum at the wrist. This condition is often associated with pregnancy, diabetes, hypothyroidism, congestive cardiac failure and inflammatory arthritis. Predisposing factors are fluid retention, local pressure on the nerve from fatty deposits and bony deformities.

Presenting signs and symptoms are paraesthesia and pain in the distribution of the median nerve (Figure 21.1), although many patients may find it difficult to localise their pain to this distribution. Pain may also radiate to the forearm and at a later stage there may be motor symptoms with wasting of the thenar eminence. Patients often complain of a sense of swelling but there is rarely any objective evidence of this. Pain is frequently worst at night.

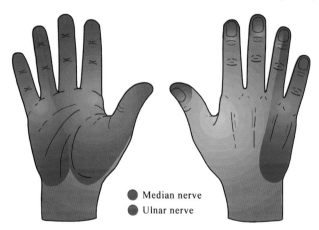

Figure 21.1
Distribution of median and ulnar nerve

● Median nerve
● Ulnar nerve

The diagnosis can be confirmed by two tests:

- Phalen's test: ask the patient to push together the dorsum of both hands with the wrists fully flexed for one minute—this should reproduce the symptoms;
- Tinel's test: percussion over the median nerve at the wrist should reproduce the symptoms.

If the diagnosis remains uncertain nerve conduction studies may be required. Management of carpal tunnel syndrome consists initially of night splints worn for a few weeks. This is often sufficient to cure mild cases. If the fluid retention is associated with obesity then weight loss may help but the use of diuretics makes no difference. If splinting alone does not solve the problem then a steroid injection into the carpal tunnel may be helpful, taking care to avoid the median nerve. If symptoms persist after injection then the patient should be referred for consideration of surgical decompression to prevent long-term numbness and muscle wasting.

TRIGGER FINGER

This can occur in the flexor tendon sheaths of any finger and is also common in the thumb. It is caused by inflammation of the flexor tendon sheath giving rise to a nodule on the tendon causing blockage to free movement of the tendon within the sheath. Classically the patient presents complaining of an inability to extend one finger actively although it can be pushed straight by the other hand. Management consists of a local steroid injection into the synovial sheath around the nodule avoiding the nodule itself and taking care not to inject into the tendon. Injection usually resolves the problem but in the few cases where it is unsuccessful, surgical release may be required.

MALLET FINGER

This condition results from a tear of the insertion of the extensor tendon from the base of the distal phalanx. (Figure 21.2) There is usually a history of injury and there may be an associated fracture, so it is usual to x-ray this injury, despite the fact that fracture or not the management is the same. Clinical features are an inability to extend the distal inter-phalangeal joint actively though it can be done passively and often there

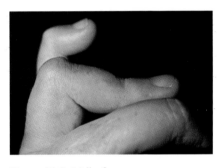

Figure 21.2 *Mallet finger*

is associated swelling and tenderness. Management consists of the application of a mallet splint, which holds the joint in full extension for six to eight weeks to allow the tendon insertion to re-attach. Rarely surgical intervention is needed.

DEQUERVAIN'S TENOSYNOVITIS

This is an inflammation of the tendon sheaths of extensor pollicis brevis and abductor pollicis longus where they run over the styloid of the radius and

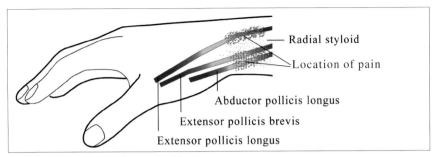

Radial styloid

Location of pain

Abductor pollicis longus

Extensor pollicis brevis

Extensor pollicis longus

Figure 21.3 *De Quervain's tenosynovitis*

below the extensor retinaculum (Figure 21.3). The sheaths become stenosed and inflamed causing pain on extension of the thumb sometimes associated with swelling and tenderness. Classically there is crepitus, which can be felt on movement of the thumb as the inflamed surfaces move within the sheath. The diagnosis can be confirmed by Finkelstein's test where the patient folds his or her thumb into the palm of the hand and makes a fist around the thumb producing passive ulnar deviation which reproduces the pain. Pain can also be elicited by resisted extension of the thumb. This condition is associated with overuse and repetitive movement. Management includes avoiding the precipitating movement, use of a resting splint, physiotherapy and ultrasound and use of anti-inflammatory and analgesic drugs. Steroid injection into the tendon sheath but avoiding the tendon itself often produces a very good result.

DUPUYTREN'S CONTRACTURE

In this condition there is thickening of the palmar fascia causing gradual fixed painless flexion of one or more fingers (Figure 21.4). The condition usually affects the ring and little fingers first. Dupuytren's contracture is associated with diabetes, high alcohol intake, family history and increasing age, and some believe it may be more common in those who have worked in heavy manual industries. Many people have mild contractures which do not cause any

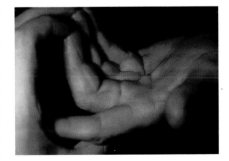

Figure 21.4 *Dupytren's contracture*

real problems but some develop significant disability which may interfere with work or leisure activities and in these patients surgical division may be warranted.

GANGLIA

These are swellings of the synovial lining of tendon sheaths or joints and occur commonly around the wrist (Figure 21.5). They are filled with a gel like fluid which may be difficult to aspirate. Ganglia often disappear spontaneously but frequently recur. If aspiration is unsuccessful surgical removal may be required.

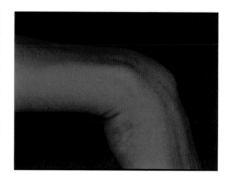

Figure 21.5 *Ganglion at the wrist*

chapter 22

Hip problems

OSTEOARTHRITIS OF THE HIP

Osteoarthritis is one of the most common causes of pain around the hip. The pain is usually insidious but may present and deteriorate fairly rapidly. Classically pain is felt in the groin or antero-lateral thigh but hip osteoarthritis may also present with pain in buttock. The first and most sensitive measure of hip osteoarthritis is internal rotation of the hip which is tested by flexing the hip and knee to 90° and rotating the hip internally and externally using the lower leg as a pointer (Figure 22.1). Other signs of hip osteoarthritis which may be present include shortening of the leg and wasting of the gluteal muscles.

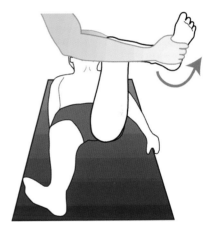

Figure 22.1 *Testing hip rotation*

Differential diagnoses of hip osteoarthritis

These include:

- hernia;
- pelvic pathology;
- referred pain from knee or lumbo-sacral spine;
- trochanteric bursitis;
- metastatic lesions.

There are three main soft tissue problems occurring around the hip.

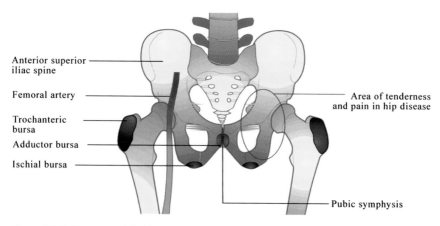

Anterior superior
iliac spine

Femoral artery

Trochanteric
bursa

Adductor bursa

Ischial bursa

Area of tenderness
and pain in hip disease

Pubic symphysis

Figure 22.2 *Bursae round the hip*

Trochanteric bursitis

The trochanteric bursa lies over and posterior to the greater trochanter in the lateral aspect of the thigh (Figure 22.2). Inflammation of this bursa causes pain especially when lying on the side in bed. Pressure on this area in a normal person causes some mild tenderness and if inflammation is present this whole area becomes ex-tremely tender. Trochanteric bursitis is often associated with osteoarthritis. If the condition is mild sometimes local heat is all that is required but if moderate to severe it usually responds to a steroid injection into the bursa. If necessary the injection may be repeated after a few weeks.

Ischial bursitis

This is much less common than trochanteric bursitis and causes pain over the buttock at the ischial tuberosity (Figure 22.2). This pain is often worse when the patient is sitting on a hard surface. On examination there is tenderness over the ischial tuberosity when the patient is prone. If the condition does not respond to local heat and analgesia a steroid injection may be given into the ischial bursa.

Adductor tendonitis

This may occur in athletes and in patients with osteoarthritis and sero-negative spondylitis such as ankylosing spondylitis. The patient complains of pain in the inner part of the groin or thigh. There is tenderness over the insertion of the adductor tendon (Figure 22.2) and pain on resisted adduction of the leg. Conservative treatment with rest from precipitating activities, heat physiotherapy and analgesics usually solves the problem but if it persists a steroid injection into the enthesopathy may resolve the problem.

chapter 23

Knee problems

Many problems occurring around the knee especially in older age groups are due to osteoarthritis of the knee. Pain from osteoarthritis of the knee is usually felt in the anterior or medial aspect of the knee and the upper part of the tibia. If pain is worst going up or down stairs this is usually due to patello-femoral osteoarthritis. Knee osteoarthritis may be associated with a popliteal cyst.

Other conditions causing knee pain include:

- soft tissue problems around the knee may be caused by ligaments, bursae, cysts or tendons;
- referred pain from hip;
- mechanical derangement within the knee joint e.g. meniscal problems;
- inflammatory conditions;
- gout and pseudogout;
- rarely malignancy;
- knee pain conditions associated with adolescence.

SOFT TISSUE PROBLEMS

Collateral ligament strain

The collateral ligaments of the knee are very strong structures lying laterally on each side of the knee joint (Figure 23.1). Strain of these ligaments is usually associated with injury. Signs are localised pain at the insertion of the ligament, and pain which is aggravated by stressing the joint medially or laterally. Management is rest, support to the joint and if necessary a steroid injection to the point of maximal tenderness.

CRUCIATE LIGAMENT DAMAGE

Damage to the cruciate ligaments (Figure 23.1) often occurs with twisting injuries such as those sustained during sporting activities. Patients sometimes present acutely with a swollen knee due to a haemarthrosis. More minor tears may present with a history of locking and episodes of the knee giving way and

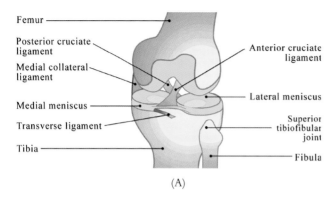

Femur

Posterior cruciate ligament

Medial collateral ligament

Medial meniscus

Transverse ligament

Tibia

Anterior cruciate ligament

Lateral meniscus

Superior tibiofibular joint

Fibula

(A)

Figure 23.1
Ligaments and menisci of the knee

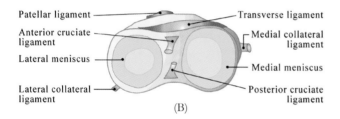

Patellar ligament

Anterior cruciate ligament

Lateral meniscus

Lateral collateral ligament

Transverse ligament

Medial collateral ligament

Medial meniscus

Posterior cruciate ligament

(B)

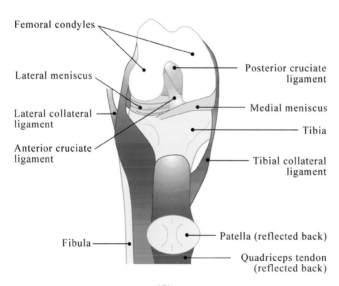

Femoral condyles

Lateral meniscus

Lateral collateral ligament

Anterior cruciate ligament

Fibula

Posterior cruciate ligament

Medial meniscus

Tibia

Tibial collateral ligament

Patella (reflected back)

Quadriceps tendon (reflected back)

(C)

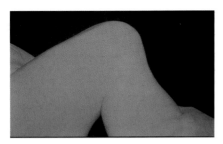

Figure 23.2 *Drawer test*

intermittent swelling. Often there is little to be found on clinical examination in chronic cases other than some effusion. It is possible to test for instability of the knee using the drawer (Figure 23.2) or Lachman test but the reliability of this test is relatively poor in the hands of a non-expert. Joint line tenderness is present in most cases of cruciate ligament problems but may also be present in other conditions so is not diagnostic. Pain increasing at the limits of extension and flexion may also suggest a cruciate ligament injury. If the history suggests a meniscal problem the patient should be referred for an orthopaedic opinion.

There are a number of bursae around the knee but those most commonly giving problems are the prepatellar, the infrapatellar and the anserine (Figure 23.3).

PREPATELLAR BURSITIS

Otherwise known as 'housemaid's knee' this condition is usually related to repetitive minor trauma and occurs in those who lean down and forwards on a knee repeatedly in the course of their daily work such as joiners, carpet layers etc. The wall of the bursa becomes thickened, an effusion develops within the bursa and the whole area over the front of the patella often looks red and shiny (Figure 23.3). The redness is usually due to inflammation rather than infection although these bursae sometimes do become infected and this may need to be excluded. The condition usually resolves spontaneously and if the bursa is aspirated it generally fills up again quickly. If conservative management is unsuccessful aspiration followed by a steroid injection may resolve the problem. Patients should be advised to use a thick foam pad to kneel on to prevent recurrence.

INFRAPATELLAR BURSITIS

The other name of this condition is 'clergyman's knee' (Figure 23.3) and again relates to repetitive minor injury this time caused by kneeling in the upright position. The patient generally complains of pain on kneeling and there is tenderness deep to the patellar tendon. Management is as for prepatellar bursitis.

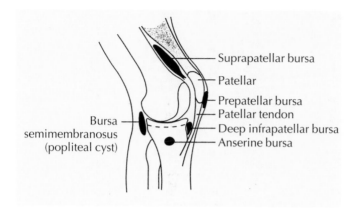

Figure 23.3
Bursae around the knee

ANSERINE BURSITIS

This is 'cavalryman's knee' (Figure 23.3) and is caused by the inner upper part of the lower leg sustaining repeated injury. This condition is associated with osteoarthritis of the knee and may be aggravated by malalignment and deformity of the knee due to the underlying osteoarthritis. Quadriceps exercises to build up the strength of the muscles may help to relieve the pressure and a steroid injection into the bursa is often very helpful.

POPLITEAL (BAKER'S) CYST

This cyst accumulates at the back of the knee in the popliteal fossa (Figure 23.4). Such cysts usually communicate with the knee joint. Patients often complain of an aching feeling and some difficulty in bending the knee. If the cyst ruptures it generally tracks down into the calf muscle and causes considerable pain due to the irritation of the synovial fluid on

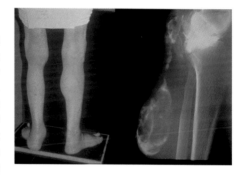

Figure 23.4 *Baker's cyst, right knee and arthrogram showing Baker's cyst*

the muscle fibres. A ruptured cyst may be difficult to differentiate from a deep vein thrombosis and may require an ultrasound scan to be sure of the diagnosis. A ruptured cyst is usually treated by a steroid injection into the knee joint.

chapter 24

Ankle and foot problems

The foot is a rather neglected area in rheumatology and orthopaedic teaching and yet foot problems are a common reason for consultation in primary care.

Many foot problems are due to structural deformities such as loss of the transverse or longitudinal arch or 'pes cavus', or claw foot. Other problems are due to generalised or systemic conditions such as rheumatoid arthritis, sero-negative spondyloarthropathies, osteoarthritis, gout or diabetes. Some conditions such as bunions (hallux valgus) (Figure 24.1) may be aggravated by ill-fitting or inappropriate footwear. Pain in the forefoot may be due to 'Morton's neuroma' a condition where the interdigital nerve becomes trapped causing neuralgic type pain frequently between the third and fourth toes.

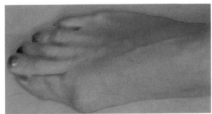
(a)

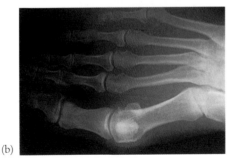
(b)

Many foot conditions can be relieved by using suitable footwear, such as impact absorbing soles and by using devices such as arch supports. Surgery may be required for treatment of hallux valgus and neuromas. If simple devices and suitable footwear do not resolve the problems referral to a podiatrist may be helpful for provision of a specific orthotic device. If the foot pain is due to a systemic cause then obviously the underlying condition should be treated.

Figure 24.1 (a) *Hallux valgus,* (b) *x-ray of Hallux valgus*

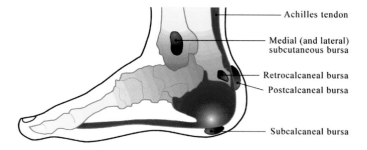

Achilles tendon

Medial (and lateral) subcutaneous bursa

Retrocalcaneal bursa

Postcalcaneal bursa

Subcalcaneal bursa

Figure 24.2
Bursae of the foot and ankle

There are a number of soft tissue conditions which occur around the foot and ankle due to bursitis (Figure 24.2), tendinitis and enthesopathy.

RETROCALCANEAL BURSITIS

The retrocalcaneal bursa lies deep to the Achilles tendon and inflammation of this bursa gives rise to ankle pain worse on exercise and relieved by rest. There is usually tenderness lateral to the Achilles tendon. Conservative treatment is usual with rest and analgesics and anti-inflammatory drugs if needed. It is possible to inject steroid into the bursa but great care must be taken to avoid injection into the Achilles tendon as tendon rupture may occur with medico-legal implications.

POSTCALCANEAL BURSITIS

The postcalcaneal bursa lies over the Achilles tendon just above its insertion into the calcaneus. Bursitis here gives pain on running and there is tenderness over the bursa. There is often a history of wearing a new pair of shoes. Rest and avoidance of the precipitating factor generally solves the problem.

ACHILLES TENDINITIS

The patient presents with pain and tenderness over the tendon. There is often some diffuse swelling and there may be crepitus on movement. Pain is exacerbated by using the tendon such as when standing on one's toes. In this condition a steroid injection is contraindicated because of the danger of causing a rupture of the tendon. Symptoms are usually treated by rest and anti-inflammatory drugs although if these measures are unsuccessful a plaster cast may be required to immobilise the tendon.

TIBIALIS POSTERIOR SYNDROME

This condition is due to inflammation of the tibialis posterior tendon and sheath. These structures lie behind the medial malleolous and may become inflamed in athletes and sportspeople and sometimes in inflammatory arthropathy. The patient complains of medial ankle pain and on examination there is an elongated tender swelling in the region of the tendon which is exacerbated by rolling beneath the fingers. This condition often responds to a steroid injection into the tendon sheath but it is a technically difficult procedure and the patient is best referred to a specialist

PLANTAR FASCIITIS

This condition is due to inflammation of the attachment of the plantar fascia to the calcaneum (Figure 24.3). It is also known as 'policeman's heel' and is common in those people who walk a lot on hard surfaces in non-shock absorbing footwear. Symptoms are of poorly localised heel pain worse on walking. Examination often demonstrates tenderness on deep pressure to the sole of the foot over the plantar fascia attachment. Treatment is initially using a heel pad to absorb impact. If this unsuccessful a course of ultrasound can be

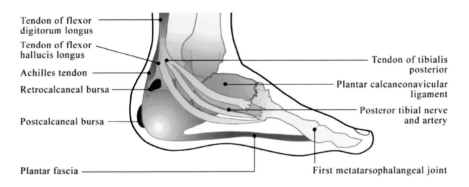

ARTICULAR PAIN	PERIARTICULAR PAIN	REFERRED PAIN
Hallux valgus	Bunion	Posterior tibial nerve
Osteoarthritis	Retro- and post- calcaneal bursa	
Inflammatory arthritis	Achilles tendinitis	
Gout	Plantar fasciitis	
Infection	Ligamentous injuries	

Figure 24.3 *Sources of pain in the foot and ankle*

very helpful. The condition also often responds to a steroid injection into the point of maximum tenderness. As the skin on the sole of the foot is thick and hard such an injection is often rather unpleasant for the patient if given through the plantar aspect and is much less painful if given from the medial aspect.

REFERRAL

Consider referring patients with:

- foot problems due to systemic diseases;
- suspected Morton's neuroma;
- hallux valgus for consideration for surgery;
- mechanical foot problems for podiatry assessment and orthosis;
- tibialis posterior syndrome and retrocalcaneal bursitis for steroid injection;
- Achilles tendinitis if not settling with symptomatic treatment;
- plantar fasciitis for ultrasound or steroid injection.

chapter 25

Knee pain in an adolescent

Teenagers often present to primary care with a history of knee pain. This can be due to a number of different conditions:

- trauma;
- osteochondritis dissecans;
- Osgood–Schlatter disease;
- anterior knee pain syndrome;
- chondromalacia patellae.

TRAUMA

Acute trauma is usually obvious from history and examination. If there is any instability in the joint or an acute effusion which is suspected to be a haemarthrosis the patient should be referred immediately to hospital for an orthopaedic opinion.

Chronic trauma on the other hand may give rise to some of the conditions listed below.

OSTEOCHONDRITIS DISSECANS

This usually occurs in 15 to 20 year olds who present with a history of knee pain with locking and swelling and the knee giving way. It is due to a small piece of bone from one of the condyles becoming detached and forming a loose body within the joint (Figure 25.1). X-ray may confirm the condition but direct referral is required for arthroscopy and washout to remove debris.

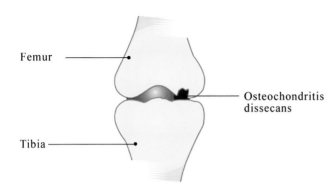

Figure 25.1 *Diagram showing site of damage in Osteochondritis dissecans*

Femur

Osteochondritis dissecans

Tibia

OSGOOD-SCHLATTER DISEASE

This condition tends to occur in boys aged 10 to 16 years who are keen footballers or athletes. They present with pain at the front of the knee and sometimes the history suggests that the pain started while actually taking part in activity. The underlying condition is inflammation at the attachment of the patellar tendon to the tibia. There is usually pain, tenderness and swelling over the tibial tubercle (Figure 25.2). X-rays are unhelpful and not required and there is no need to refer. Treatment (usually unpopular with the patients!) consists of avoiding running, kicking and other similar activities for a period of around six months.

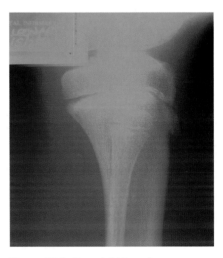

Figure 25.2 *Osgood-Schlatter disease*

ANTERIOR KNEE PAIN SYNDROME

This condition is also due to over-activity in athletic pursuits but is more common in teenage girls. Pain is the main symptom and is worse on going up or down stairs and on sitting with knees bent. X-rays are unhelpful but

MRI or arthroscopy may reveal fissuring and degenerative signs in the cartilage on the underside of the patella. If this is the case the condition is known as chondromalacia patellae (see below).

Anterior knee pain can be very difficult to treat and may last for months and even years. Girls should be advised to avoid high-heeled shoes and to use trainers or some other form of impact absorbing insoles. Physiotherapy to strengthen the muscles around the knee joint can be helpful and strapping is also sometimes used. Athletic activity is best avoided initially until the severity of the condition is assessed and analgesics or even NSAIDs may be required in the short term.

CHONDROMALACIA PATELLAE

This condition is diagnosed on arthroscopy where the underside of the patella shows fissuring. Trimming of any loose cartilage from the back of the patella together with a joint washout to remove debris is sometimes undertaken but often the results are disappointing.

REFERRAL

An adolescent with knee pain should be referred immediately with:

- acute joint instability;
- haemarthrosis;
- acute meniscal injury;
- suspected fracture

and referred routinely with:

- history of locking.

Referral should also be considered for a patient with anterior knee pain which is lasting for several months and which has failed to respond to conservative management.

Part 4

OPTIONS FOR MANAGEMENT

chapter 26

Patient education and self-management

One of the most effective ways of improving the confidence and coping abilities of patients in relation to their disease is to provide education, information and back-up support. This can be achieved in many different ways depending on staff and facilities available and also on patient preference. Education and support strategies include:

- written information;
- audiotape or video;
- face to face discussion;
- telephone contact and review;
- group education;
- individualised management plans written in conjunction with the patient;
- interactive computer programmes;
- Internet information;
- self-help groups;
- patient support organisations;
- self-management programmes.

If written information is given it is not sufficient simply to provide the information and to send the patient away to read it on his/her own, assuming that he/she will, in fact, read and understand the content. Some patients are put off by written information while others may not understand the content but are reluctant to admit this or to return to ask for clarification. Even if the patients do read and understand the information, they may not retain important facts and most will require to have advice reiterated and emphasised. It is therefore the responsibility of all healthcare professionals continually to provide education and information to our patients, and during the course of a long chronic disease such as arthritis, we have ample opportunities for this. Within primary care, as we often see our patients at regular intervals, we can educate them a little at a time and constantly provide back-up of this information and education as part of our routine consultation.

Particularly with lifestyle measures of weight loss and exercise, which are important in the management of osteoarthitis, back pain etc, it is vital to provide continual encouragement and support to enable patients to become involved in their own self-management and thus improve the long term outlook. Increasingly there are facilities available from local authorities and through health boards for patients to take part in exercise schemes to improve general fitness and we, as health care professionals, should play our part in this by encouraging our patients to become involved as appropriate and to make suitable exercise a part of their daily or weekly routine. With weight loss it is also very important to provide regular back-up and support as most patients find it very difficult to change eating habits that have been established over many years.

Around the country there are many different patient education programmes available that have been specifically developed to meet the needs of the local population. Most of these target patients with rheumatoid arthritis although some are also available for osteoarthritis. Some patients benefit from attending self-help meetings run by groups such as the Pain Society and Arthritis Care. Arthritis Care also co-ordinates a self-management programme for rheumatoid arthritis and osteoarthritis patients. This is based on a programme developed by Dr Kate Lorig at the University of Stanford in the USA. Several studies have demonstrated the long term effectiveness of the programme which is run by trained volunteers all of whom themselves suffer from arthritis.

The programme, called 'Challenging Arthritis', aims to provide:

- motivation;
- confidence-building;
- setting and achieving goals;
- advice about working with health professionals to get the most out of the treatment available.

The course consists of six weekly sessions each lasting about half a day, and is accompanied by a book.

Many arthritis patients have found great benefit from the course not only from the practical aspects but also in diminishing the sense of isolation often experienced by arthritis sufferers.

Contact details are available in Appendix 2.

chapter 27

Physical therapy

INTRODUCTION

The GP often refers patients directly to the physiotherapist, or the referral may be dealt with via the rheumatologists. There are many initiatives under way to fast track patients by a means of rapid referral to physiotherapy whenever possible. The purpose of this chapter is to highlight some of the priorities of the physiotherapist in the methods of assessment and treatment which will enable the patient to access physiotherapy as early as possible. This chapter will give an insight into the area of physiotherapy and its various treatment initiatives in some of the common diagnoses.

The rheumatology physiotherapist is a specialist practitioner who often deals with the following diagnoses in broad categories including:

- rheumatoid arthritis and inflammatory arthritis;
- spondyloarthropathies;
- connective tissue diseases;
- systemic lupus erythematosus (SLE);
- localised soft tissue rheumatism;
- low back pain/cervical pain;
- crystal arthritis.

RHEUMATOID ARTHRITIS

The physiotherapist should be involved in the early management of the patient. In many units the physiotherapist is able to fast track the patient to the most appropriate areas for assessment and treatment. This may be in the community, at home, in a health centre, or perhaps in the hospital where access to splinting, hydrotherapy, education groups and, in some places, rehabilitational gymnasium classes with emphasis on aerobic fitness. There is a definite change in emphasis with such a patient and where possible the aim must be to help maintain the patient's current hobbies and activities. The current research is to evaluate cardiovascular fitness and the patients ability to exercise.

Assessment

This should include subjective and objective measures: the measurement of joint range, muscle power, upper and lower limb function, pain management, mobility and exercise tolerance. The physiotherapist often use goniometry, Oxford scale, VAS, Ritchie articular index, HAQ, and HAD questionnaires. For an example of a rheumatoid arthritis assessment, see Table 27.1.

The physiotherapist must assess all aspects of physical, emotional and social wellbeing.

Physiotherapy management of rheumatoid arthritis

The physiotherapist is often working in an expanded role and often acts as an extended scope practitioner . Following on from the initial assessment, a programme must be formulated for the individual. There are currently various systems looking at the overall management. On an in-patient basis this may be looking at early supported discharge whereby the patient spends less time in hospital if an integrated care plan (ICP) is provided and nursing and paramedical input is given at home supporting the patient and family/carer. Another model is an outreach service referred to as Rapid Response Rheumatology (RRR). The GP has immediate access to the therapist by helpline or immediate referral. This should enable the patient, particularly when in a flare, to have appropriate treatment immediately. This would involve a home visit or priority, i.e. next day visit to the hospital clinic. The therapist would assess and implement a fast track programme often involving hydrotherapy, individual out-patient treatment, education/counselling, or access a specialised clinic e.g. joint injection clinic. The physiotherapists have extended their role to provide joint injections after appropriate training in conjunction with the Chartered Society of Physiotherapy Guidelines.

Treatment interventions

Orthotics Orthotic treatment of hand disease in patients with rheumatoid arthritis focuses on rehabilitation and splinting, with the evaluation of hand function with emphasis on grip strength and assessment of grips i.e. pinch, power, precision. Orthotics are used in various stages as a means of preventing deformity. Studies of orthotic use are limited due to lack of well controlled studies (see Table 27.2 for examples).

Table 27.1 *Example of a rheumatoid arthritis assessment*

Physiotherapy Database   **Set up date:**

GP name and address	Patient label
Tel No:	Tel No:
Consultant:	Occupation:
Rheumatology diagnosis:	Extra-articular manifestations:

Past medical history   **Joint surgery (Year)**
Cervical instability/insufficiency........................   ...Upper limbs................lower limbs................
Respiratory dysfunction...
Unstable cardiac condition.....................................
Hypertension..
Angina / MI...
(N)IDDM...
Epilepsy..
Osteoporosis...
Anaemia..
CVA..   ...General surgery...................................
Renal impairment...
Recent DVT / PE..
Incontinence..
Other..

Previous medication (Rheumatology) - no longer taken:

Imaging

Social circumstances: Smoker: cpd   Alcohol   upd

Lives with:

Type of house: Stairs: Internal: Bannisters
                               External: Bannisters

Cooking / cleaning / shopping done by: patient / spouse / family / friend / H.H   dpw

Mobility: Indoors:
            Outdoors:

Transfers: (specify)

HAQ Score:

Date: Physiotherapist:

Physiotherapy Assessment   **Admission date:**

Current medication	Patient label

Presenting complaint (Reason for admission)	Patient view of current problems

Body chart - pain / stiffness

EMS:

R   L

PAIN
1. Mild   R = Replacement
2. Moderate
3. Severe

ROM and power assessment

			Comments and power (Oxford scale)
Cervical Spine			
F	LR	LSF	
E	RR	RSF	
Shoulders	R	L	
F			
ER(HBN)			
IR(HBB)			
Elbows	R	L	
F			
E			
PRO			
SUP			
Wrists	R	L	
F			
E			
Hands	R	L	
Grip Range			
Opposition			
Hips	R	L	
F			
E			
ABD			
ER			
IR			
Knees	R	L	
F			
E			
Stability			
Ankles	R	L	
DF			
PF			
Subtalar			

Supplies: Collar   WHS   RHS   TENS

Observations and standing posture:

Date: Physiotherapist:

Physio Assessment

Physiotherapy Problem List	Intervention	Plan	Tx	CTx	Date/Sign
Systemic inflammatory pain	Cryocuff				
Local inflammatory pain	Hotpack				
Mechanical pain	TENS				
	Acupuncture				
	Hydro				
Decreased ROM	Ex programme				
General muscle weakness / deconditioned	Quads drill				
Specific muscle weakness	Ward ex class				
Instability / Hypermobility	Collar				
Decreased hand function	WHS				
Decreased UL function	RHS				
Decreased LL function	Knee splint				
Metatarsalgia	Insoles				
	Malleoloc				
	Other				
Bed mobility					
T/F Lying to Sitting	T/F practise				
T/F Sit to Stand	Walking aids				
T/F Bed to Chair / Chair to Chair	Zimmer				
Standing balance	Rollator				
Gait	Fisher stick(s)				
	Mobilisation				
	Other				
Stairs	Stair practise				
Other	Surgical appl				
	Podiatry				
	OT referral				
	HAV				
	Other				

Comments:

Physiotherapist: Date:

Discharge summary:

Discharge Plan:

OP PT referral ☐   Rehab class ☐   Podiatry ☐   Home ex programme ☐

OP Hydro ☐   Education group ☐   Surgical appl ☐   Other ☐

Physiotherapist: Date:

Table 27.2   Orthotic use

Cervical Spine:	• collars – advise day and night use • exercises	– moulded collar (atlantoaxial/subluxation) sublaxial – soft collar
Shoulder:	• use of sling for support • resting positions	– arm held in adduction with a body strap and elbow in flexion
Elbow:	• air jet splint – to stretch elbow contracture • resting position mid range of flexion	– applied daily for 1 hour to gently stretch. – moulded splint/backslab made to measure by therapist.
Hip:	• skin traction to reduce hip pain, often overnight	– to distract joint.
Knee:	• valgus knee brace • serial plaster of paris to correct flexion deformity • night resting splint	– valcro brace with hinges to give med/lat stability – moulded backslab or universal splint
Ankle:	• talcocral joint – ankle foot orthosis • subtalor joint – heel cup, malleoloc • footwear	

Exercise

The therapist must fully assess the patient, assessing their physical ability and if medically stable a starting point for exercise. A programme should include muscle strengthening, range of movement exercise and more emphasis on cardiovascular (aerobic) exercise. Testing procedures may include e.g. a ten metre Shuttle walk test: this involves a set course with a distance whereby the patient is also timed over ten metres. (See S.J. Singh, M.D.L. Morgan, A.E. Hardman, C. Rome and P.A. Barobley, 'Comparison of oxygen uptake during a conventional treadmill test and shuttle walking test in chronic airflow limitation' *European Respiratory Journal* 1994; 7: 2016-20.)

Figure 27.1   Neck and upper limb problems

RA ASSESSMENT

SUMMARY OF DEFORMITIES

1   **Neck Pain**   pain, soft collar, moulded collar and
                                advice
    Cervical myclopathy   neurological signs – ,moulded collar
    RA neck disease   assess gait, activities of daily living

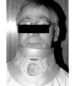

Neck Pain

2. **Glenohumeral Assessment of Joint**
    acromio-clavicular/subacromial bursa
    glenohumeral
    scapulothoracic movement
    rotator cuff
    shoulder girdle–flexion, adduction and medical rotation

3. **Elbow joint**
    loss of extension
    fixed flexion deformity
    loss of supination

4. **Wrist**
    volar subluxation
    flexion
    radial deviation

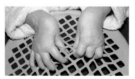

Wrist

5. **Hand**
    volar subluxation
    flexion
    ulnar deviation
    Boutonniere/Swan neck deformities

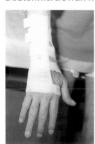

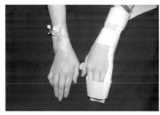

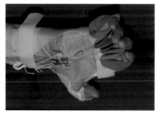

Hand-resting night splint

Dynamic splint following MCP joint
replacement

Working daytime
splint

Figure 27.2 Lower limb problems

1. **Hip joint**
   fixed flexion/adduction/lateral rotation
   extensive exercises–lying prone
   prevent flexion deformity–hip traction
   shock absorption in the feet (insoles)

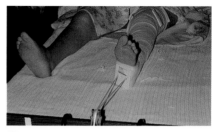

Skin traction

2. **Knees**
   Valgus and flexion deformities
   – quadriceps exercises
   – progressive stretching
   – specialized spinting

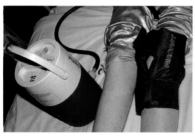

Cryotherapy for synovitis

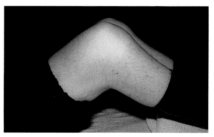

fixed flexion deformity of the knees

3. **Ankles/feet**
   valgus deformity

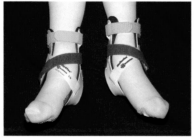

Subtalar joint malleoloc (support and correct)

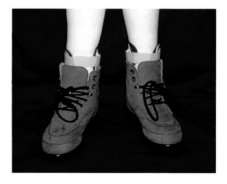

Appropriate specialised footwear

Hydrotherapy

There are various research projects to assess the benefits of this therapy. This is an ideal environment for exercise, especially when the patient has a flare of disease. The therapist gives exercise to mobilise, strengthen and introduce aerobic types of exercise in a controlled, progressive manner involving most of the affected joints. This facility helps promote early ambulation and intensive rehabilitation in an in-patient or out-patient setting.

Ice/heat

Ice: cryotherapy is often advised in the management of pain and home treatment is often recommended. Heat: during remissions this can be helpful in reducing muscle spasm.

Gait analysis

Gait re-education is often a priority in maintaining independence and in providing joint protection. There are special walking aids available for the rheumatoid arthritis patient, e.g. Fischer sticks with a moulded handle to improve the grip for the patient.

Transcutaneous electrical nerve stimulation (TENS)/acupuncture

TENS and acupuncture are used widely in the management of rheumatoid arthritis. TENS is useful as an adjunct to treatment and this can help the patient manage their pain as this often varies in different joints, especially during an acute flare.

Acupuncture is a useful adjunct to treatment and can be helpful for specific areas where muscle spasm is evident, especially in the spine. This can be helpful in facilitating exercise when there is a loss in range of movement.

Education

It is particularly helpful after diagnosis to have a programme of education involving all the multidisciplinary team. This involves discussions on medication, exercise, pain management and relaxation, diet, social work issues, podiatry, occupational therapy and involvement of voluntary organisations. In the management of arthritis the aim of this course is to empower the patient to deal with their own of care and therefore seek help or advice from the appropriate professional/organisation (e.g. Arthritis Care).

Osteoarthritis

The therapist often deals with osteoarthritis affecting the hip, knee and spine.

Osteoarthritis of the knee

The patient with osteoarthritis of the knee has pain in and around the knee. This is often exacerbated when weight bearing and improved with rest. There is often a degree of morning stiffness, crepitus on movement and a reduction in range of movement. On assessment it is important to consider any peri-articular disorder such as an infrapatella, suprapatella or ansenine bursitis.

Physiotherapy treatment

This includes:

- exercise : a muscle strengthening regime of quadriceps musculature in the form of a specific programme of isometric, isotonic and resistive exercises;
- gait: use of a walking aid, i.e. stick, if indicated;
- biomechanical assessment of feet, often involving shock absorption in the form of heel inserts;
- strapping, in the form of a medial patellofemoral strapping;
- knee brace: this is occasionally required if there is tibiofemoral disease complicated by lateral instability;
- function: advice regarding function and exercise tolerance is often helpful in encouraging the patient to remain active and maintain a level of aerobic fitness. This may take the form of a conditioning programme involving swimming or hydrotherapy.

Osteoarthritis of the hip

The principles of managing the knee also apply to the hip. The prevention of a flexion contracture and preservation of internal and external rotation are paramount. An individual assessment is made assessing pain, range of movement, muscle power, function and aerobic fitness. The therapist often gives heel pads for shock absorption and checks for a leg length discrepancy. All of these factors are extremely important in preserving function and independence.

Osteoarthritis of the spine

There are several highly trained back therapists who provide a thorough assessment and management programme for osteoarthritis of the spine. They often offer individual treatment, access to back school and groups with emphasis on ergonomics, moving and handling and conditioning programmes. It is of paramount importance to maintain activity with emphasis on early movement and function, not long term bed rest. There are always local initiatives and national initiatives ongoing throughout the United Kingdom.

Surgical intervention

If the patient requires surgery, it is essential that they attend for a pre-assessment by a therapist to prepare for the operation, maximise their function pre-operatively and receive their conditioning programme, in order to facilitate a good outcome. This can help reduce their length of stay in hospital.

ANKYLOSING SPONDYLITIS

The physiotherapist has a primary role in the management of patients with ankylosing spondylitis by optimising their exercise therapy, with emphasis on strengthening, maintaining full range of movement and aerobic fitness. A detailed annual assessment of the axial skeleton is documented and targets identified in the form of goals. In most areas of the country there are local groups organised as National Ankylosing Spondylitis Support Groups. They often meet weekly and have group exercise sessions in a gymnasium and in many areas a hydrotherapy/swimming pool. The emphasis is on conditioning and aerobic fitness. The patient is encouraged to facilitate his own personal home programme of exercises and activities. In some patients a detailed assessment of function is indicted, including assessment of driving.

A maintenance programme is important and it is the therapist's role to

Table 27.3 Areas affected by enthesitis

	Treatment
• C7/T1	Advice on movement/acupuncture/TENS
• stenoclavicular joint	Ultrasound/exercise
• stenocostal joint	Ultrasound/injection
• iliac chest	Ultrasound/injection/stretch exercise
• hip adduction origin	Ultrasound/injection
• greater trochanter	Ultrasound/injection
• insertion of plantar fascia	Ultrasound/acupuncture/shock absorption
• Achilles tendon	Ultrasound/acupuncture/shock absorption

motivate these patients to exercise—this is the key to preserving function and overall aerobic fitness. Early assessment is highly recommended for these patients. Treatment of an enthesitis is important as this quickly limits function. Enthesitis often affects the areas shown in Table 27.3.

Treatment

The management of an enthesitis varies but local treatment consisting of ultrasound, cryotherapy, exercise, including stretching and mobilising, is often indicated.

Posture Re-education of posture is essential, therefore preventing deformities. Patients with this condition classically adopt the posture with a flattening of the lumbar spine, a kyphosis and a poking chin as they protract their cervical spine.

Pain Pain often reduces with exercise and a reduction in stiffness. A TENS machine can be useful for self-management of pain.

Individual programme A programme should include the following:

- warm up;
- stretches (e.g. pectorals, hamstrings);
- mobilising exercises (neck rotation);
- strengthening (back extensions);
- aerobic activities (exercise bike);
- flexibility (trunk side flexion);
- balance, co-ordination, proprioception (ball games);
- function (pelvic tilt);
- warm down.

The therapist and patient should agree on certain goals and methods for quickly checking the patient's range of movement.

SYSTEMIC LUPUS ERYTHEMATOSUS (SLE)

Patients with SLE demonstrate a non-erosive arthritis, symmetrical and commonly affecting knees, wrists and hands. Contractures and deformities are usually a result of soft tissue problems and joint subluxation. Tenosynovitis is often evident and there is occasional rupture of tendons. There is often some degree of myalgia. Patients often have a reduced exercise tolerance and complain of fatigue. An assessment of muscle power as a baseline is important and a graduated conditioning programme given with definite reviews organised.

SYSTEMIC SCLEROSIS

The therapist should consider the patient's respiratory function, range of movement with attention to contractures and likely pressure areas, when considering how active a rehabilitation programme should be. It is important to give active exercise with a conditioning element incorporating aerobic and stretching exercise. A holistic approach should include a relaxation programme.

DEMATOMYOSITIS AND POLYMYOSITIS

The assessment of a patient with this condition should include a detailed muscle chart at presentation and during flares to determine the exercise and often functional support that may be required for facilitating activities of daily living, e.g. stairs. A gait assessment is important and a waddling gait is often demonstrated due to proximal weakness in the lower limbs. The stage of inflammation should be recognised and the patient provided with home support and open access to physiotherapy when it is required.

SPONDYLOARTHROPATHIES

These conditions comprise:

- psoriatic arthritis;
- enteropathic spondyloarthropathy;
- reactive arthritis;
- Reiters syndrome;
- ankylosing spondylitis.

A physiotherapist assessment is often the same as for rheumatoid arthritis. The spine is often affected and care should be taken to assess specific limitation in movement. An approach as for ankylosing spondylitis should be adopted.

SOFT TISSUE RHEUMATISM

The therapist commonly deals with various problems which include local areas and other conditions such as fibromyalgia and hypermobility syndrome. Effective treatments should include stretching, strengthening, and muscle balancing techniques. The key to successful management of a soft tissue lesion is in accurate diagnosis, therefore appropriate management and this

Table 27.4 Common soft tissue problems

Upper limb

Shoulder

Acute or chronic capsulitis	ice/passive or active movements/ injection
Acromioclavicular joint acute or chronic capsulitis	mobilising exercise/taping/injection
Sternoclavicular joint acute or chronic capsulitis	exercise /injection
Supraspinatus tenponitis	ultrasound/exercise/frictions/injection
Infraspinatus tendonitis	ultrasound/exercise/frictions/injection
Subscapularis tendonitis or bursitis	exercise/injection
Subdeltoid bursitis	exercise/injection

Elbow joint

Acute or chronic capsulitis	range of movement exercise/injection
Common extension origin , 'tennis elbow'	deep frictions/ultrasound/injection
Common flexor tendon, 'golfer's elbow'	deep frictions/ultrasound/injection
Biceps tendon insertion , tendonitis or bursitis	frictions/ultrasound/injection/exercise
Olecranon bursa	injection

Wrist joint

Acute capsulitis (RA)	injection/splint/active movement

Lower limb

Hip

Acute capsulitis	injection/re-education movement/gain re-education
Adductor tendonitis	deep friction massage/injection
Ishcial bursitis	injection/exercise
Global bursitis	injection/exercise
Psoas bursitis	injection/exercise
Trochanteric bursitis	injection/exercise

Knee

Capsulitis	aspiration/injection/exercise/re-educate movement
Superior tibiofibular joint	injection
Coronary ligament	deep friction/injection
Medial collateral ligament	ice/massage/mobilisation/injection
Quadriceps expansion	deep friction/injection
Infrapatellar tendonitis/bursitis	deep friction/taping/injection/graded exercise
Pes ansenine bursa	injection/stretching
Ilotibial band bursa	injection/rest/stretch
Baker's cyst	aspirate/culture/re-educate movement

Ankle

Subtalor joint/mid tarsal joint	injection/active movement
Capsulitis	injection/re-educate movement
Achilles tendon	deep friction/injection

may also involve a local steroid injection. The Chartered Society of Physiotherapy has guidelines for chartered physiotherapists, who have been giving injections since 1995. A summary of some of the soft tissue lesions are listed in Table 27.4.

chapter 28

Pharmacological therapy

Although drug therapy is only one part of the management of musculo-skeletal problems it is nevertheless an extremely important part. Most patients with musculo-skeletal problems will at some time be treated with drugs. This may be for:

- symptom control;
- prevention of long term damage;
- reducing or modulating inflammation.

In this section we will examine all the categories of drugs used in the management of musculo-skeletal problems and consider their indications, pharmacology, side effects and interactions as well as dosing regimes. The groups of drugs we will consider include:

- analgesics;
- topical agents;
- non steroidals (NSAIDs);
- coxibs;
- disease modifying anti-rheumatic drugs (DMARDs);
- biological agents;
- drugs used in the management of gout;
- corticosteroids;
- muscle relaxants.

Sometimes one drug alone will be used but more commonly patients with significant problems will be taking several different drugs, e.g. a 73 year old female patient with severe rheumatoid arthritis may be taking DMARDs together with NSAIDs and analgesics for symptom control, a drug to treat her osteoporosis, and a gastro-protective agent to avoid complications from her NSAID therapy.

Many patients with rheumatological conditions are in the older age groups and many will be suffering from other diseases and taking concomitant medication for these conditions. It is important for all those prescribing to review patient's drug therapy at regular intervals to avoid unnecessary prescribing with its problems of interactions and side effects. It is also sensible to try to reduce the number of drugs taken in an attempt to avoid confusing elderly patients who can become very mixed up about their medication especially if they live alone. Dosette boxes with spaces for tablets to be placed in separate compartments corresponding to different dosage times throughout the day may be a good aid to compliance. These boxes may be filled by the patient's relatives but it is usually more satisfactory for the pharmacist to fill the boxes on a weekly basis.

Another danger for the prescriber is that sometimes new symptoms are treated with additional medication which is then added to the repeat prescription system. Any new symptom should be assessed in conjunction with a review of the current drug therapy, as it may be one of the currently prescribed drugs which is causing the problem. The solution then would be to alter the current medication either by stopping it, by reducing the dosage or by substituting an alternative.

Computer-generated repeat prescription systems are in use in most GP surgeries. While they can save much work and can help in audit etc. they can lead to drugs being put on to the repeat system, sometimes without full evaluation of the results. These drugs are then continued perhaps inappropriately. Similarly when a patient is discharged from hospital, an immediate discharge letter detailing current drug therapy usually accompanies them. It is important to check the patient's drug record at this time as the new drugs may be added to the existing repeat prescribing list already on the computer, causing considerable confusion for the patient. For these reasons it is very important to have regular reviews of each patient's medication.

Computer-generated systems are immensely useful in highlighting any potentially dangerous co-prescription of drugs as most modern systems have some kind of warning to alert the prescriber of an inappropriate combination of medication.

PRACTICE POINTS

Remember to:

- regularly review repeat medication;
- avoid unnecessary prescribing;
- consider dosette boxes to aid compliance.

ANALGESICS

Analgesics are widely used in all musculo-skeletal problems. Increasingly many analgesics can be bought from the pharmacy, although the stronger analgesics still require a doctor's prescription. Simple analgesics are often all that is required in the management of conditions such as osteoarthritis, when combined with education and various lifestyle changes and intermittent analgesic therapy is by far the safest of the pharmacological options available.

Patients often require considerable education in the appropriate taking of analgesia and there are a number of misconceptions, which are widely held. For example:

- 'Painkillers only mask symptoms, I want something that treats the under-lying condition': while it is true that analgesics do not have any effect on the underlying conditions, there is also very little evidence that, for example NSAIDs have any effect on non-inflammatory conditions, other than their analgesic effect. It is important that patients should understand that sometimes analgesics are the correct way of managing certain condi-tions, such as mechanical back pain, so that not only does the analgesic reduce the unpleasant sensation of pain but also, by lessening pain, helps the patient to retain mobility and keep muscles in good condition, which is extremely important for the long term outcome.
- 'Paracetamol is dangerous': while it is true that paracetamol in overdosage is dangerous, paracetamol alone nevertheless remains one of our safest analgesic options. Many patients fail to realise that paracetamol is contained in many of the products which can be bought from a pharma-cist. Patients are often afraid to take adequate doses of paracetamol because they are concerned about the potential danger of overdose and it is impor-tant to reassure them in this regard, that it is a safe drug within the normal dosage of up to 4gm/day.
- 'If you can buy it from the pharmacist, it is not very effective': patients often present asking for stronger analgesics, as those they have tried from the pharmacist have not been effective. On further discussion, however, you may find that the patients have not been taking the drug in adequate dosage, at regular enough intervals and for a long enough period of time.
- 'I don't want to become addicted to tablets': there is no evidence that paracetamol is addictive, although patients can become dependent on opiate-based medication.

The most common analgesics used are:

- paracetamol alone;
- paracetamol with codeine or dihydrocodeine;
- paracetamol with dextropropoxyphene;
- codeine or dihydrocodeine alone.

Codeine, dihydrocodeine and dextropropoxyphene are all opiate-based and so may have some of the opiate side effects, such as constipation and addiction. Other analgesics used for musculo-skeletal pain are nefopam, meptazinol and tramadol:

- nefopam is useful in some patients particularly the elderly, for moderate pain due to a musculo-skeletal problem. It is a non-opioid preparation, chemically a benzoxazocine. It can be effective but can give sympathetic and antimuscarinic side effects;
- meptazinol is an opiate partial-agonist. It is said to have a low incidence of respiratory depression but can cause nausea and vomiting. Again it can be effective in pain of musculo-skeletal origin ;
- tramadol is an opiate analogue, with two mechanisms of action. It has an opiate effect and also enhances serotoninergic and adrenergic pathways and in theory gives fewer opioid side effects. It can be an effective and fairly strong analgesic but can cause some psychiatric reactions.

TOPICAL PREPARATIONS

Topical preparations are commonly used for minor musculo-skeletal problems and for many patients they will be the first choice prior to seeking medical help. They can be particularly helpful in minor injuries such as strains and sprains and in osteoarthritis of the small joints of the hand and sometimes in osteoarthritis of other areas such as elbow, wrist and ankle. There is some doubt as to the mechanism of action of these topical preparations and it may be that any benefits are due to the process of rubbing, acting as massage, rather than the actual substance rubbed on. There are, however, several studies, which show a benefit to using a topical agent over placebo, where both are being rubbed on. Another benefit of a topical agent, which is sometimes forgotten, is that all topical therapies give patients a degree of control over their own condition, and psychologically this can be extremely valuable. Three groups of topical preparations are available:

Rubs or embrocations

These products seem to work by producing counter-irritation of the skin. This stimulates the sensory nerves, which then compete with the pain signals produced by the affected area, resulting in a decrease in the pain message transmitted to the brain from the affected area.

Some preparations, such as capsicum, salicylates and nicontinates, contain rubefacients, which produce vasodilatation giving a feeling of warmth, while others such as camphor or menthol give a sensation of coolness. These products have been available for many years and there is little evidence to support their use. Some patients, however, find them helpful and they are not only cheap but also very safe and can be used in conjunction with other therapies.

Topical NSAIDs

A number of NSAIDs have been produced in a cream, foam or gel form suitable for rubbing over an affected area. These preparations are considered by many doctors to be expensive and no more effective than rubs or embrocations and for these reasons are rarely included in drug formularies. It has been shown, however, that therapeutic levels of the active drug can be found in the synovial fluid and surrounding tissues after use but without the high serum levels obtained after oral dosing, thus reducing systemic side effects. A recent meta-analysis (Moore *et al*, BMJ, 1998) has shown that some topical NSAIDs can be effective in treating both acute painful conditions, such as soft tissue trauma, sprains and strains, and also chronic pain conditions including osteoarthritis and tendinitis. Results suggest that around one in three patients achieve 50% reduction in pain over and above the effect of placebo, with the number needed to treat 3.9 for acute conditions and 3.1 for chronic conditions.

Although side effects of topical NSAIDs are not common, they should not be prescribed to patients in whom there is a contraindication to oral NSAID therapy, as there is some systemic absorption.

Capsaicin

Capsaicin is a topical cream made from hot chillies. The rationale for its action is that it depletes substance P, which is a neuropeptide involved in the transmission of pain in the afferent nerve fibres. Substance P is thought to stimulate synoviocytes to produce prostaglandins and collagenases, and levels of substance P are raised in inflamed joints. Studies have shown a gradual decrease in osteoarthritis pain, with the maximum benefit experienced after around four weeks of therapy. Capsaicin cream has to be applied four times a day, as a very small bead, and has some practical disadvantages in that the patient may have to remove clothing such as tights to apply the cream at these regular intervals. The main side effects of this therapy are stinging or burning sensations experienced by around 40% of patients. It is important to wash hands immediately after application to avoid contact with sensitive body areas, such as the eyes. In clinical practice most patients improve over the first few weeks of treatment.

Capsaicin has been used in the USA for over ten years and the American College of Rheumatology suggests its use for osteoarthritis of the knee as the next stage in pharmacological therapy, following paracetamol.

NON STEROIDAL ANTI-INFLAMMATORY DRUGS

Non steroidal anti-inflammatory drugs (NSAIDs) are used very commonly and probably over prescribed in primary care. They have an anti-inflammatory effect and also some analgesic effect. Patients often prefer to take an NSAID rather than an analgesic in the misguided belief that the drug is somehow treating their arthritis. It is true, however, that many patients, with what appears to be a non inflammatory condition such as osteoarthritis, seem to gain benefit from an NSAID as it may give better symptom control than an analgesic, in particular where stiffness is a problem. Dosage regimes for NSAIDs are usually simpler than for analgesics and many are given only once per day, thus aiding compliance. NSAIDs however have considerable problems with side effects, and interactions and care should be taken when prescribing one of these drugs.

The most serious problems associated with NSAID prescription are perforations or bleeds from an NSAID-induced peptic ulcer. It is estimated that as many as 2600 people die each year in the United Kingdom from the above complications, that is one in every 1200 patients prescribed an NSAID. Although these numbers are considerable many GPs will not themselves see many patients with such problems and may underestimate the potential problems associated with NSAID prescription.

Mode of action of NSAIDs

In 1971 Sir John Vane suggested that NSAIDs work by inhibiting the biosynthesis of prostaglandins, which lead to the development of inflammation. It was eventually realised the NSAIDs inhibit the enzyme cyclo-oxygenase (COX), which leads to the production of inflammatory prostaglandins.

In 1991 it was discovered that there were two isoforms of cyclocygenase (COX). (Figure 28.1)

■ COX 1 constitutive (or housekeeping) which leads to the production of prostacyclin, protecting the gastric mucosa, prostaglandin E2, protecting kidney function and thromboxane A protecting platelet function.

■ COX 2 inducible (or inflammatory) form, which leads to the production of proteases, prostaglandins and other inflammatory mediators giving rise to inflammation. It has recently been found, however, that COX 2 also has a constitutive role in maintenance of kidney function and probably also in other physiological functions.

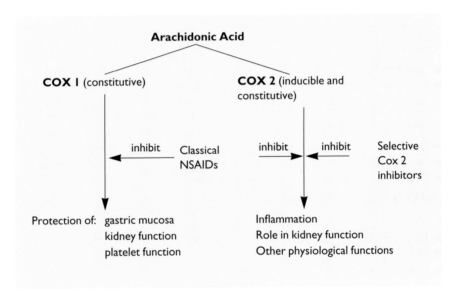

Figure 28.1 *Site of inhibition of classical NSAIDs and selective COX 2 inhibitors*

As classical NSAIDs inhibit both COX 1 and COX 2 activity, while they are effective in decreasing inflammation, they may lead to the loss of gastric and renal protection.

In theory an ideal NSAID would be one which blocked the development of inflammation, while, at the same time, preserving gastric protection and renal and platelet function. This would then reduce inflammation, while leaving the physiological protective mechanisms intact, so reducing gastric, renal and platelet side effects.

Limitations to NSAID use

Oral NSAIDs have a number of side effects, contraindications and interactions.

NSAID side effects

Gastro-intestinal:

- Perforation of ulcer
- Bleed from peptic ulcer
- Dyspepsia
- Nausea
- Diarrhoea
- Iron deficiency anaemia from chronic gastro-intestinal bleeding
- Colitis

Renal side effects:

- Renal failure
- Interstitial fibrosis
- Papillary necrosis

Hypersensitivity reactions:

- Rash
- Bronchospasm
- Angio-oedema

CNS Side effects:

- Tinnitus
- Photosensitivity
- Headache
- Personality change

Fluid retention also occurs and this may precipitate heart failure especially in the elderly

In 1994 the Committee for the Safety of Medicines (UK) reported on the relative safety of saveral NSAIDs in terms of serious upper GI side effects (Table 28.1). All those included were so called classical or standard NSAIDs with no selective effect on COX 2. Azapropazone is no longer used as a routine NSAID and has restrictions on its prescribing imposed by the CSM. NSAIDs in the intermediate group continue to be used although there is greater use of the lower risk drug ibuprofen, which is available from pharmacies without a doctor's prescription.

Table 28.1 NSAID risk groups

Lowest risk	Ibuprofen
Intermediate risk	Diclofenac
	Indomethacin
	Naproxen
	Ketoprofen
	Piroxicam (at higher end of intermediate group)
High risk	Azapropazone

The CSM report did not include several newer drugs, such as etodolac, meloxicam and nabumetone, all of which appear to have some selective COX 2 inhibition. These drugs seem to give rise to less gastric side effects than the classical NSAIDs.

Contra-Indications to NSAIds

- Active peptic ulceration.
- Pregnancy and lactation.
- Haemophilia.
- Aspirin or NSAID allergy.
- Angioneurotic oedema.

Relative Contra-Indications to NSAids

Cases where NSAIDs are best avoided but may be used with special care if absolutely necessary:

- Past history of peptic ulceration or gastrointestinal bleed.
- Current dyspepsia.
- Asthma.
- Renal impairment.
- Congestive cardiac failure.
- Hypertension.
- Hepatic impairment.
- Warfarin therapy.

Interactions

NSAIDs have a number of interactions some of which apply to all NSAIDs as a class effect, while others may only apply to a particular drug. The main class interactions include anticoagulants, diuretics, lithium, methotrexate, quinolone antibiotics, oral hypoglycaemics, ACE inhibitors and betablockers. Individual NSAIDs may also interact with cyclosporin, hydantoins and digoxin.

Special Precautions

Elderly patients, smokers and those on long term oral steroids are at highest risk of developing gastro-intestinal complications of NSAID therapy. Elderly patients are more likely to suffer from conditions where NSAIDs may cause problems, such as renal failure, or be taking concomitant medication, such as ace inhibitors or digoxin, giving greater potential for interactions. If NSAIDs are thought to be necessary for an acute inflammatory flare or for pain control where other measures have failed, they should be prescribed at the lowest dose and for the shortest time possible.

Co-Prescription

In a patient taking a classical NSAID who is at risk of developing a gastro-intestinal side effect, preventive therapy with misoprostol, ranitidine or proton pump inhibitors may be given. Misoprostol reduces serious gastro-intestinal side effects by around 40% but may cause indigestion and diarrhoea. Routine co-prescription of misoprostol does not appear to be cost effective. Ranitidine is licensed to prevent duodenal ulceration and proton pump inhibitors, though more expensive, are licensed for the treatment and prophylaxis of NSAID ulceration, both gastric and duodenal, and are usually well tolerated.

COX-2 Inhibitors

Recently there has been considerable interest in drugs which selectively block COX 2. COX-2 inhibitors with a high degree of selection include rofecoxib and celecoxib and are sometimes known as COX-2 specific blockers or coxibs. Some NSAIDs previously available such as meloxicam, etodolac and nabumetone have been found to have varying degrees of COX 2 selectivity, greater than that found in classical or standard NSAIDs.

COX-2 selective inhibition appears to reduce the potential for serious gastro-intestinal side effects although this effect is reduced in patients taking low dose aspirin. COX-2 selective inhibitors also do not appear to have an antiplatelet effect and in patients with cardio-vascular disease, standard NSAIDs may be safer from the cardiac viewpoint. Both COX 1 and COX 2 seem to have a role to play in the maintenance of renal function and inhibition of COX 2 may cause similar renal side effects to standard NSAIDs.

If a patient is at high risk of developing a gastro-intestinal side effect and requires NSAID therapy, prescription of a selective COX-2 inhibitor should be considered. Such patients would include those with a past history of gastro-intestinal problems, those taking concomitant medication such as corticosteroids, those with serious co-morbidity, those requiring long term high dose therapy and those in the older age groups.

DISEASE MODIFYING ANTI-RHEUMATIC DRUGS (DMARDs)

DMARDs are drugs which have an effect on the long term outcome of rheumatoid arthritis, and other inflammatory arthritides not only in terms of symptoms by reducing pain, swelling, stiffness and improving general wellbeing but also in terms of prevention as they have been shown to have an effect in reducing radiological changes and thus helping to prevent joint deformities.

In the past DMARDs were used at a later stage of disease, when many long term problems had already been established. In the last few years, however, several studies have shown that the early introduction of DMARDs can help to prevent long term problems and improve both functional and radiological outcome. Current practice suggests that DMARDs should be introduced as soon as possible in the course of the disease and preferably as soon as rheumatoid arthritis is diagnosed to try to prevent long term damage. Two further randomised-controlled studies against placebo showed that withdrawal of DMARDs produced relapse and again current thinking suggests that the use of DMARDs should be long term and continuous.

DMARDs can be fairly toxic agents and most require haematological and/or biochemical monitoring. Many areas now use a shared care system, whereby patients who are established on DMARDs have drug monitoring carried out from the GP surgery, rather than at hospital outpatients. Most patients find this beneficial, as it reduces travelling time.

Most GPs now prescribe DMARDs once they have been initiated at hospital and are also responsible for monitoring. It is, therefore, important that GPs are aware of the side effects, interactions and monitoring requirements for all these drugs, as the responsibility for the drug lies with the person prescribing, i.e. the GP who is signing the prescription. Most rheumatological departments will send the GP a copy of the monitoring requirements when they initiate a new DMARD and many also operate a telephone helpline, where the primary care team can receive advice about side effects, changes in blood parameters etc.

Some GPs may initiate therapy with a DMARD following a telephone consultation with the consultant rheumatologist prior to the patient being seen at outpatients, particularly if there is going to be a considerable delay in this appointment and thus a delay in therapy. This would normally only happen with a GP who was experienced and confident in the initial diagnosis of rheumatoid arthritis, and this diagnosis is not always easy in the early stages of disease.

It is extremely important that those practitioners undertaking drug monitoring for DMARDs set up a system to check that patients receive regular monitoring and that the blood results are read by someone with an understanding of the monitoring requirements. Often it is not sufficient simply to look at the fact that the levels are within normal values because an increasing or decreasing trend may be important, for example a decrease in white cell count over time or an increase in alkaline phosphatase levels. Changes such as these, while still within the normal range, may indicate a developing problem and it is important to read the monitoring results in a continuum.

The most commonly used DMARDs for patients with recently diagnosed and active rheumatoid arthritis are sulfasalazine and methotrexate. These two drugs have been shown to have probably the best efficacy/toxicity trade off. Hydroxychloroquine and auranofin seem to have less efficacy than other DMARDs. Hydrocycholoroquine in particular is often used for less aggressive rheumatoid arthritis, as it tends to have fewer side effects and requires no blood monitoring. It may also useful in the early stages of disease, when the actual diagnosis of an inflammatory arthritis may be uncertain.

Patients on DMARD therapy should be warned to report immediately if they develop a sore throat, unexplained bleeding, mouth ulcers, fever, purpura or rash as these may be associated with a blood dyscrasia.

Sulfasalazine

This drug has been around for many years and as well as being used as a DMARD for inflammatory arthritis it is also used extensively for inflammatory disease of the bowel.

Chemical structure The drug is a combination of 5-aminosalicylic acid and sulfapyridine available in 500mg enteric coated tablets.

Uses It is used to treat rheumatoid arthritis, psoriatic arthritis and reactive arthritis.

Dosage schedule 500mg/day for one week increasing by 500mg/day each week until a maintenance dose of 2.5 to 3 gms is reached.

Onset of action Onset takes six to ten weeks.

Side effects
- nausea with dose increases (this can be treated by prochlorperazine);
- skin rash (which can sometimes be treated by desensitisation) in which the patient receives a very small dose of the drug initially with gradual increments over weeks and months until a therapeutic dose is reached. This may prevent the reappearance of the rash enabling the patient to continue with the drug;
- diarrhoea, headache, mouth ulcers, reversible oligospermia and staining of soft contact lenses;
- neutropenia, leucopenia, thrombocytopenia may occur in the first three to six months of treatment and are usually reversible on stopping the drug;
- abnormal LFTs.

Interactions
- decreases the absorption of digoxin;
- interacts with warfarin and phenytoin.

Contraindications
- best avoided during pregnancy but may be used if essential. There is a theoretical risk of neonatal haemolysis in third trimester, and the mother should take adequate folate supplements;
- excreted in breast milk giving the theoretical risk of neonatal haemolysis;
- should not be used in men wishing to father a child because of the possibility of oligospermia although it is important to note that it is not an effective contraceptive.

Monitoring FBC and LFTs should be taken at the start, then FBC twice weekly and LFTs four times weekly for 12 weeks, then three-monthly for a year, then six monthly thereafter.

Methotrexate

This drug is an immunosuppressant.

Uses It is used to treat rheumatoid arthritis and other inflammatory diseases.

Dosage It is given as a once weekly oral dose usually starting at 7.5mg/week increasing if necessary to 15-20mg/week depending on response. Increases in dose are usually given at intervals of six weeks. Lower doses of 5mg/week may be sufficient in frail elderly patients or those with renal impairment. It may be given intramuscularly or subcutaneously if required.

Side effects
- relatively common side effects such as skin rash, alopecia, nausea and diarrhoea;
- less commonly leucopenia, thrombocytopenia and liver cirrhosis;
- rarely pneumonitis in patients with rheumatoid arthritis and patients should be advised to contact a doctor immediately if they develop dyspnoea or cough;
- folic acid 5mg taken three days after each dose of the drug helps to reduce toxicity.

Interactions
- trimethoprim and co-trimoxazole, increasing the anti folate effect;
- penicillins and NSAIDs, reducing excretion;
- cyclosporin, retinoids and probenecid.

Contraindicationss:
- the drug is teratogenic and contraindicated in pregnancy and lactation, and conception should be avoided for at least six months following administration;
- it may also affect both male and female fertility;
- administration of live vaccines is contraindicated during therapy.

Monitoring Pre-treatment FBC, LFTs and renal function tests and chest x-ray should be carried out. Thereafter, FBC weekly until six weeks after the last dose increase and then monthly. LFTs should be checked every two to four months and U&Es every six to 12 months.

Hydroxychloroquine
This drug is anti-malarial.

Uses It is used to treat rheumatoid arthritis, other inflammatory arthritis, and connective tissue disease but should not be used for psoriatic arthritis.

Dosage The usual starting dose is 200mg twice daily but some patients require only 200mg/day or 200 to 400mg on alternate days.

Side effects:
- can rarely cause retinopathy but this is unlikely provided the recommended dosage is not exceeded. Screening recommendations from the Royal College of Ophthalmologists suggest that patients starting hydroxychloroquine should have a baseline eye check by an optometrist and if any abnormality is detected patient should be referred to an ophthalmologist.

It is often difficult to distinguish drug-induced retinopathy from age-related macular degeneration. Patients should be asked to report any changes in visual acuity;
- can cause rash and gastrointestinal upset;
- can be very toxic in overdosage.
- headache.

Interactions:
- amiodarone;
- anti-epileptic drugs , reducing anti-convulsant effect;
- digoxin, increasing plasma digoxin concentration;
- cyclosporin, increasing cyclosporin concentration;
- antacids, which should not be given concomitantly as they reduce the absorption of the drug.

Contraindications The drug is contraindicated in pregnancy.

Monitoring Apart from baseline renal and liver function tests to determine any dose adjustments, no blood monitoring is required.

Intramuscular gold
This treatment uses sodium aurothiomalate.

Uses It is used to treat rheumatoid arthritis and psoriatic arthritis.

Dosage It is administered by deep intramuscular injection. A test dose of 10mgs is given and following this, 50mgs/week until clinical signs and symptoms improve. It is usual to see some benefit when around 300 to 500mgs in total dose has been given, although it may require up to 1gm in total before there are signs of remission. If no benefit is seen at a total dose of 1gm, the therapy should be discontinued. Once there are signs of a clinical response, intervals between injections should be gradually increased from weekly to every four weeks, although if there are any signs of relapse, the dose can once more be increased to weekly.

Side effects
- skin rashes, mouth ulcers;
- nephrotoxicity and pancytopenia;
- more severe reactions, which occur in up to 5% of patients.

Interactions
- nephrotoxic drugs;
- immunosuppressant drugs.

Contraindications
- should not be used if there is any history of severe kidney or liver problems or blood disorders;
- is contraindicated in pregnancy and lactation as it has been shown to cross the placenta and to be teratogenic in animal studies. It is excreted in breast milk but very little appears to be absorbed by the baby, although there is a theoretical possibility of rashes and idiosyncratic reactions – probably best avoided in lactation.

Monitoring FBC tests and urinalysis should be carried out at baseline and prior to each injection.

Leflunomide
This drug is an immunosuppressant, broken down in the body to an active metabolite, which persists over a very long period.

Uses It is used to treat active rheumatoid arthritis.

Dosage The usual dose is 100mgs/day for the first three days, reducing to a maintenance dose of 10-20mgs/day.

Side effects
- diarrhoea;
- alopecia;
- hypertension;
- nausea.

Interactions
- live vaccines, which are contraindicated during immunosuppressant therapy.

Contraindications
- the drug is contraindicated in pregnancy. Because of persistent levels of active metabolite, women who have leflunomide treatment should not conceive for at least two years following discontinuation of the treatment. For men who receive leflunomide treatment there should be a gap of at least three months between stopping treatment and attempting conception. This long waiting time can be reduced with special washout procedures, which are also needed if serious adverse effects occur or if another DMARD is to be started (Table 28.2);
- because leflunomide acts as an immunosuppressant there is a theoretical increase in risk of infection and malignancy;

Table 28.2 Washout procedure for leflunomide

- Stop treatment
- Give either cholestyramine 8gm tid for 11 days or activated charcoal 50gm qid for 11 days
- Conception should not be attempted until the concentration of the active metabolite has been shown to be less than 20mcg/litre(measured twice 14 days apart)

- the drug should not be given if there is liver impairment or any evidence of serious infection.

Monitoring Liver transaminases and blood pressure should be checked at baseline and regular intervals afterwards. FBC, including differential white count and platelets, should be checked at baseline and then two weekly over first six months of treatment and eight weekly thereafter.

Azathioprine

This drug is an immunosuppressant.

Uses It is used to treat rheumatoid arthritis and psoriatic arthropathy in patients who have failed to respond to the more commonly used DMARDs. Sometimes used in conjunction with corticosteroid therapy to try to reduce the dose of corticosteroids, producing a corticosteroid sparing effect.

Dosage 1.5 to 2.5mgs/kgm/day in divided doses. The dose should be reduced in the elderly.

Side effects:
- nausea, vomiting and diarrhoea often occur early during the course of treatment and may necessitate stopping therapy;
- leucopenia can occur;
- because azathioprine is an immunosuppressant, there may be an increased risk of infection.

Interactions:
- warfarin;
- co-trimoxazole and trimethoprim;
- allopurinol;
- ACE inhibitors;

- live vaccines, which are contraindicated during immunosuppressant therapy.

Contraindications The drug is contraindicated where there is hypersensitivity to mercaptopurine or azathioprine.

Monitoring FBC should be checked weekly for first four weeks, thereafter three monthly. LFTs should be checked monthly for three months.

Auranofin

This is an oral gold preparation, less commonly used than intamuscular gold.

Uses It can be used to treat rheumatoid arthritis, although it is less effective than intramuscular gold, sulfasalazine, penicillamine and methotrexate.

Dosage 6mgs/day initially which can be increased to 9mgs/day after six months.

Side effects Diarrhoea and others side effects similar to intramuscular gold.

Contraindications Similar to intramuscular gold.

Monitoring Similar to intramuscular gold.

Penicillamine

This is a penicillin derivative which acts in a similar way to gold.

Uses It is used to treat rheumatoid arthritis.

Dosage 125mgs/day for the first four weeks, increasing by 125mgs at minimum intervals of four weeks up to 500mgs/day after six months of treatment. The dose can then be increased, if required, by 125mgs, again every four weeks, up to 750mgs/day after 36 weeks and eventually, again by 125mgs every four weeks, up to 1 gm/day.

Onset of action It takes up to 12 weeks to bring about any improvement.

Side effects:
- nausea;
- rash;
- proteinuria;
- pancytopenia;
- loss of taste, which usually returns a few weeks later irrespective of whether or not the drug is stopped.

Interactions Iron, antacids and zinc can all decrease the absorption and therefore reduce the effect of the drug.

Contraindications The drug is contraindicated during pregnancy and lactation.

Monitoring FBC, urea, electrolytes tests and urinalysis should be carried out at baseline, then urinalysis weekly and FBC two weekly until dose is stable, thereafter FBC and urinalysis four weekly. It is also advisable to check FBC count two weeks after any dose increase.

BIOLOGIC AGENTS FOR RHEUMATOID ARTHRITIS

Recently some new biologic agents for the treatment of rheumatoid arthritis have become available. The ones at present available, etanercept and infliximab, are tumour necrosis factor (TNF) alpha antagonists. These drugs appear to be very effective in rheumatoid arthritis and in a recent study combining infliximab with methotrexate, there was found to be virtually no radiological progression. This appeared to occur with or without a clinical response. This is obviously very important because if radiological progression can be stopped and hence the structural damage reduced, this will have a number of long term benefits, both clinical and economic.

The two drugs at present available are:

■ etanercept, which is a recombinant human TNF receptor:Fc fusion protein. It is administered subcutaneously at a dose of 25mgs twice weekly;

■ infliximab; which is a chimeric human-murine monoclonal antibody administered by slow intravenous infusion every four to eight weeks at a dose of 3-10mgs/kg. Infliximab is usually given in combination with oral methotrexate.

These treatments are new and very expensive. At present there is insufficient long term data to justify their use across the board in patients with rheumatoid arthritis. Eventually in the United Kingdom they will be used in accordance with the British Society for Rheumatology Guidelines, which include:

■ a standardised measurement of disease activity indicating highly active disease;

■ failure of standard therapy, including adequate therapeutic trials of at least two standard DMARDs, of which methotrexate should be one.

One of the problems with these drugs is the fact that they may aggravate infection. They should, therefore, not be given to patients who have active infection or are at high risk of infection, including patients with chronic infective conditions such as leg ulcers, previous septic arthritis, bronchiectasis, Mycobacterium Tuberculosis, indwelling catheters etc. They should also not be given in pregnancy, lactation or to patients with malignant disease.

Initially these drugs will potentially be used in patients with more severe rheumatoid arthritis, who have failed conventional therapy. This would produce both a clinical and economic benefit.

It is anticipated that all patients prescribed these therapies in the United Kingdom should be registered centrally so that data on progression and side effects can be monitored at a central level. These drugs will, of course, only be initiated in secondary care for some time but it may be that GPs who have patients with rheumatoid arthritis not attending secondary care should re-refer such patients for consideration of anti-TNF alpha therapy. If these drugs prove to be as effective as anticipated, the future of patients with rheumatoid arthritis will be transformed.

Rheumatoid arthritis is an enormously expensive disease. It has costs:

- to society, in terms of loss of work by patients;
- to the National Health Service, in terms of drug costs;
- in disease modifying agents;
- in analgesics and NSAIDs;
- in other necessary drugs, such as osteoporosis therapy, gastro-protection and antidepressants;
- in patient consultations, in both primary and secondary care;
- in spells of inpatient treatment;
- in therapist treatment for physiotherapy and occupational therapy;
- for monitoring DMARDs.

Although TNF alpha receptors can be expensive, if they can effectively stop the longer term process of rheumatoid arthritis, they may well be extremely cost effective.

DRUGS USED IN THE MANAGEMENT OF GOUT

Acute attacks

Acute attacks of gout are most often treated with NSAIDs in fairly high doses, unless there is a contraindication to the use of these drugs. If so, colchicine is the drug of choice. It is as effective as NSAIDs but can give rise to toxicity in higher doses. Unlike NSAIDs it can be used in patients receiving anti-coagulants and also in patients with heart failure as it does not cause fluid retention. Colchicine is given as a dose of 1mg initially followed by 500mg every two to three hours until either pain is relieved or nausea or diarrhoea occur. A total dose of 6 mg is the maximum within any three-day period. Colchicine should not be given to patients receiving cyclosporin therapy.

Prevention

If acute gout occurs on more than one occasion it is worth then considering some preventive therapy. Prevention can be undertaken by two methods:

- by decreasing the formation of uric acid from purines;
- by increasing the excretion of uric acid by the kidney.

The most commonly used drug is allopurinol, a xanthine-oxidase inhibitor, which reduces the formation of uric acid. It is usually fairly well tolerated and treatment should be continued in the long term. It is usually given in a dose of 100–300mgs/day depending on the severity of the condition and the plasma uric acid levels. Lower doses of the drug, 100mgs/day, are often sufficient to control uric acid levels, especially in elderly patients, but in patients with more severe conditions 700-900mgs/day may be required. Side effects include rash and hypersensitivity reactions. Allopurinol can be used in patients with renal impairment. It may interact with ACE inhibitors, anti-coagulants, cyclosporin and azathioprine.

Uricosuric agents increase the excretion of uric acid. The two drugs in this group are probenecid and sulfinpyrazone. Both these drugs can be used as alternatives to allopurinol but are generally less well tolerated and should be avoided in patients with renal impairment or urate stones. Both drugs may lead to crystallisation of urate in the urine. To avoid this a good fluid intake of at least 2 litres per day should be taken especially in the first few weeks of therapy. Probenecid is given in a dose of 250mg twice daily after food, increasing after one week to 500mg twice daily. Doses up to 2 gms/day may be required to reduce uric acid levels although this can often be reduced for maintenance. Sulfinpyrazone is given initially in a dose of 100-200mg daily increasing up to 600mg/day according to serum uric acid concentrations. Again this dose can usually be reduced for maintenance. Probenecid has interactions with NSAIDs, methotrexate, ACE inhibitors, antibacterials, antivirals and chlorpropamide while sulfinpyrazone has interactions with anticoagulants, sulfonylureas, phenytoin and theophylline.

When any of these preventive treatments are initiated they may precipitate an acute attack of gout. For this reason either an NSAID or colchicine should be given at the start of treatment and continued for at least one month.

CORTICOSTEROID THERAPY

Corticosteroids can have a very potent effect in reducing inflammation and are used as therapy in a number of inflammatory and connective tissue diseases. Low doses of corticosteroids are sometimes used in rheumatoid arthritis but may cause significant problems with long term morbidity (see Chapter 6, Rheumatoid arthritis). Corticosteroids are used as the main treatment in polymyalgia rheumatica and temporal arteritis and in connective tissue disorders such as systemic lupus erythematosus, dermatomyositis etc. In all conditions it is sensible to use the lowest possible dose, and to decrease the dose as soon as possible. Where there has been prolonged therapy and in potentially relapsing disease corticosteroids should be withdrawn gradually. The dose can be reduced fairly rapidly to 7.5mg/day but should then be reduced slowly over a much longer time to avoid adrenal insufficiency, which may have serious results.

Contraindications
Corticosteroids should be used with care and caution in those with:

- hypertension;
- recent myocardial infarct;
- liver and kidney impairment;
- cardiac failure;
- glaucoma;
- severe affective disorders;
- epilepsy;
- peptic ulceration;
- hypothyroidism;
- pregnancy and breast-feeding.

Side effects
Corticosteroid therapies have a number of serious side effects:

Gastrointestinal problems, including :
- peptic ulceration;
- pancreatitis;
- candidiasis.

Musculoskeletal effects including:
- myopathy;
- osteoporosis, leading to fractures;
- tendon rupture.

Endocrine effects including :
- duodenal suppression;
- amenorrhoea;
- irregular menstrual bleeding;
- hirsutism;
- weight gain.

Neuro-psychiatric effects including :
- euphoria;
- dependence;
- depression;
- psychosis;
- aggravation of epilepsy and schizophrenia.

Ophthalmic effects including:
- development of cataract;
- glaucoma;
- papilloedema.

Skin side effects including:
- skin atrophy;
- increased bruising;
- development of striae;
- impaired healing.

All patients should be informed about these side effects, prior to receiving treatment and should be given a steroid card to carry. This card should indicate patient and doctor details, specific drug taken and the dosage.

Patients with rheumatoid arthritis are more likely to have osteoporosis due to their rheumatoid arthritis and, therefore, treatment with corticosteroids may significantly increase their osteoporosis risk. Patients who are treated with steroids because of polymyalgia or temporal arteritis tend to be in the older age groups and are possibly more likely to be at risk of osteoporosis. In these patients it is useful to have a DEXA measurement at the start of corticosteroid treatment. The National Osteoporosis Society Guidelines suggest that if the steroid dose is going to continue at 7.5mgs for a period of six months or more, then the patient should be started on anti-osteoporosis therapy, such as a bisphosphonate.

Drugs available

Corticosteroid drugs available are:

■ prednisolone in oral tablets of 25mgs, 5mgs, 2.5mgs and 1mg;
■ deflazacort as oral tablets of 1mg, 6mg, and 30mg.

Sometimes drugs such as azathioprine are used to give a steroid sparing effect. This means that the same control of inflammation can be achieved, with a reduction in the dose of steroids due to the effect of azathioprine.

Interactions

Corticosteroids have important interactions with antibiotics, anticoagulants, antiepileptics, antifungals and cyclosporin, and also with a number of drugs in other categories.

Patients on corticosteroid therapy may have increased susceptibility to infection. Some infections can also be masked by steroid therapy and may reach an advanced stage before diagnosis. It is also thought that corticosteroid therapy can reactivate some latent diseases, such as tuberculosis.

Patients receiving corticosteroid therapy are at increased risk of severe chicken pox, which may not manifest itself with a typical rash but may lead to severe lung and liver infection. Once a patient on corticosteroid therapy is exposed to chicken pox, their immunity should be checked and if they are not immune, they should receive passive immunisation, preferably within three days and certainly before ten days from exposure. If a patient on corticosteroid therapy does develop chicken pox, steroid therapy should not be stopped and the patient should be referred immediately for specialist treatment. Measles can also cause particular problems to non-immune patients taking steroids and prophylaxis with immunoglobulin may be needed.

Corticosteroid therapy should not be given to patients with systemic infection, unless they are receiving specific antimicrobial therapy at the same time.

Intra-muscular and intra-articular steroid therapy

Intra-muscular steroid therapy is sometimes used in acute inflammatory conditions such as rheumatoid arthritis to help a patient over an acute inflammatory flare and provide a bridge until other therapies take effect. Intra-muscular steroid therapy can also be used to help the patient cope with a particular stress and to reduce symptoms for a specific short time, for example for a holiday or for a family wedding.

Preparations commonly used are:

- methylprednisolone (Depo-Medrone) in a dose of 40–120mg intramuscularly;
- triamcinolone (Kenalog) in a dose of 40mg intramuscularly.

Corticosteroid therapy can also be given intra-articularly to reduce inflammation within a specific joint. The effect of an injection usually lasts for about four to six weeks and by this time the inflammatory flare may have resolved or other measures such as DMARDs may have taken effect. In some patients the beneficial effect of an intra-articular injection may last for several months. Current practice suggests that several different joints can be injected at the same time although each individual joint should only be injected three or four times each year and at no less than four weekly intervals.

Contraindications to intra-articular steroid therapy Contraindications to intra-articular steroid injections include:

- infection in the joint: if in doubt do not inject steroid. Aspirate joint and send synovial fluid for culture;
- systemic infection;
- local skin infection;
- first 16 weeks of pregnancy;
- hypersensitivity to any ingredient including the local anaesthetic.

Diabetes, hypertension, osteoporosis and hypothyroidism are relative contraindications and the pros and cons of treatment should be carefully considered before an injection is given. Care should also be taken with patients on warfarin therapy.

Side effects to intra-articular steroid therapy Serious side effects to intra-articular steroid injections are not common. Infection is the most serious risk and if it occurs the patient may be seriously ill with a significant risk of death (sometimes quoted as a similar risk as that of patients with meningococcal meningitis). Having said that, rates of infection are extremely low at 1 in around 78,000 injections and can be minimised by careful sterile technique and single dose ampoules.

Other side effects include:

- transient flare of pain and inflammation;
- localised subcutaneous fat atrophy(minimised by careful placing of injection in deeper structures);
- transient hyperglycaemia;

- tendon rupture (if the injection is wrongly placed in the substance of the tendon);
- facial flushing;
- aseptic osteonecrosis;
- delay of menstruation or abnormal vaginal bleeding.

Preparations of intra-articular steroids There are three commonly used intra-articular preparations:

- hydrocortisone acetate 25mgs/ml (hydrocortistab);
- methylprednisolone acetate 40mgs/ml (depo-medrone);
- triamcinolone hexacetonide 20mgs/ml (lederspan).

Hydrocortisone acetate is the shortest acting and least potent and probably used more for soft tissue problems than intra-articular injections. It is also best used when injecting into a difficult area such as near a tendon in order to minimise any damage. Methyl prednisolone is medium acting and of moderate potency, while triamcinolone is longer acting and the most potent of the three. If required, local anaesthetic can be used to infiltrate the area of injection. This may, however, obscure the bony landmarks and make the injection technically more difficult. Many doctors prefer either to mix local anaesthetic with the steroid preparation (both hydrocortisone acetate and triamcinolone hexacetonide have a licence allowing this) or to use a pre-mixed preparation, such as depo-medrone with lidocaine, which is methyl-prednisolone acetate 40mgs/ml plus lidocaine 10mgs/ml. (See Table 28.3 for steroid dose for different joints.)

Table 28.3 Steroid dosages for different joints

knee	1ml
CMC joint	up to 0.5mls
AC joint	0.2 to 0.5mls
shoulder	1ml steroid plus 1-10ml of 1% Lignocaine, if appropriate
trochanteric bursitis	1ml steroid

Specific indications for corticosteroid therapy both oral and intra-articular are discussed in chapters on the specific diseases.

INTRA-ARTICULAR HYALURONANS

In a normal joint, hyaluronic acid is the component which gives synovial fluid its visco-elastic properties, which are essential for both shock absorption and lubrication. Hyaluronic acid may also have a role in joint repair and in supplying some anti-inflammatory and analgesic action.

Clinical trials have suggested that a series of hyaluronan injections can decrease the pain and stiffness of knee osteoarthritis for up to six months and have shown comparable or slightly better results than daily NSAIDs, but with fewer side effects. These products can, however, give some local reactions of swelling and pain.

Two preparations are available:

- hyaluronic acid 20mgs/2mls, given as a series of once weekly injections for five weeks;
- hylan GF20 16mgs/2mls, given as a series of once weekly injections for three weeks.

One study with hyaluronic acid compared with triamcinolone hexacetonide showed similar short term efficacy but the patients in the hyaluronic acid group had significantly less pain at six months. Further studies are awaited to see whether the use of these compounds has an impact on surgical referrals.

MUSCLE RELAXANTS

Skeletal muscle relaxants are occasionally used to help relieve muscle spasm, such as that caused with acute back pain and neck strains and should only be used in the short term and for acute problems.

Diazepam is one of the best muscle relaxants but of course as it is a benzodiazepine, it may cause sedation and other problems associated with this class of drug, such as addiction, although this is not usually a problem if the prescription is limited to a few days supply at the time of an acute muscle spasm.

Carisoprodol and methocarbamol are also occasionally prescribed, although there is little evidence to support their use. Some patients, however, do find these drugs helpful, in the acute stages of a back or neck injury, although again, they may cause drowsiness. The dose of carisoprodol is 350mgs tid, with half this dose for elderly patients. It should not be used in respiratory disease or porphyria, is contraindicated in lactation, and may cause gastrointestinal problems as well as hypotension, paraesthesia, weakness and other CNS effects. Methocarbamol dosage is 2 x 750mg qid, again with half this dose in the elderly. This drug should not be used in patients with epilepsy and is best avoided in pregnancy and lactation.

GLUCOSAMINE

Glucosamine is a normal constituent of synovial fluid and cartilage matrix. It is a complex sugar which is a derivative of natural aminomonosaccharides. Short term studies have suggested that glucosamine therapy has a positive effect on symptoms of OA and the compound is used as prescribed therapy in several countries in Europe and is available over the counter as a nutritional supplement in the UK. A recent long term study of glucosamine against placebo has shown no significant loss of joint space in the glucosamine group over a three year period compared with a progressive loss in the placebo group. There was also an improvement in symptoms in the active group and no differences in terms of safety between the two groups. These results would suggest that glucosamine has some effect in OA, not only in improving symptoms but also in modifying progression. The dose used in this study was 1500mg of glucosamine sulphate. Smaller doses may not show similar results. Glucosamine is sometimes combined with chondroitin which has a bovine origin.

Although further studies are required it would appear at present that glucosamine is safe, may improve symptoms and may also have a disease modifying effect on OA.

chapter 29

Surgery in the rheumatic diseases

SURGERY FOR RHEUMATIC DISEASES

End stage joint failure, i.e. destruction of the articular surface can result from inflammatory and non-inflammatory disease. Whilst medical treatment might delay the onset of joint failure, surgical treatment should be regarded as part of the process of management of disease, rather than failure of medical therapy. Indeed some surgeons, particularly those concentrating on upper limb disease, feel that results could be better if joints are surgically treated before they are completely destroyed. In end-stage joint disease, the joints are no longer able to function, and the symptoms are primarily mechanical rather than inflammatory with pain, loss of function, instability and deformity, being major symptoms. Crepitus is often found at this stage, resulting from bone on bone articulation in the absence of cartilage. Surgical options are two-fold, either arthrodesis (fusion) or arthroplasty generally total joint replacement. Indications for total joint replacement are the same for osteoarthritis (85% of cases) and rheumatoid arthritis (15% of cases). In general proximal joint surgery is undertaken before distal as this maximises functional improvement in the upper limb, and limits the potential element of referred pain to the knee or elbow.

Whilst awaiting surgical review and intervention, patients should be given the full benefit of conservative forms of treatment, including appropriate pain relief, splints, as well as physiotherapy and adaptation of the home environment by the occupational therapists. Intra-articular steroids can also ameliorate painful flares of synovitis in rheumatoid arthritis, and injection of hyaluronan into the knee is reported beneficial in osteoarthritis of that joint.

MEDICAL/ANAESTHETIC PROBLEMS

Patients with rheumatic disease often have significant co-morbidity and this should be taken into account at the time of surgery. Standard complications of surgery apply, and appropriate prevention methods applied. Particular problems occur in ankylosing spondylitis, where there can be difficulty with intubation because of rigid cervical spinal structure. Similarly, limitation of rib cage movement can cause poor ventilation post-operatively.

In rheumatoid arthritis bone quality is poor and post and peri-operative fracture can complicate surgery and recovery. Bone grafting may be required to support replaced joints as in the case of acetabular protrusion. Cervical spine involvement requires extra care with intubation to ensure that neck extension does not cause damage to the cervical cord. The immunosuppressive action of certain disease-modifying drugs might interfere with healing: some authors stop methotrexate and azathioprine, but data on this is minimal. Because of the polyarticular nature of rheumatoid arthritis, particular consideration should be given to pre-operative planning. It is appropriate to consider each joint in association with limb and total body function, especially as replacement surgery will be ongoing requiring rehabilitation and medical treatment between surgical interventions. The use of forearm crutches, elbow crutches or sticks can be a limiting factor in rehabilitation following lower limb surgery if there is significant upper limb disease.

SPECIFIC SURGICAL PROCEDURES

Synovectomy

Acute synovitis is painful and can be associated with local impingement (e.g. carpal tunnel syndrome) and synovial rupture (e.g., Baker's cyst of the knee). Synovectomy can improve range of movement of the flexor sheathes and prevent further tendon damage, but requires intensive physiotherapy post-operatively. The single swollen joint that fails to respond to standard medical therapy can be relieved by synovectomy, which can be undertaken through the arthroscope or as an open procedure. Synovectomy often precedes joint replacement in the longer term.

Tendon transfer

Tendon ruptures commonly present acutely with inability to move single digits in the hand. Extensor pollicis longus rupture leads to loss of active extension of the distal interphalangeal joint of the thumb, whilst extensor digitorum longus damage at the radio-ulnar joint can cause the fingers to drop with inability to extend the fingers. Repair is undertaken either by transfer of intact extensor tendons or by transplanting undamaged tendon into the ruptured site. Tendon rupture of tibialis posterior presents as a development of the progressive, painful flat foot, and Achilles' tendon rupture with acute pain in the back of the calf. If developed acutely, reconstruction is feasible but requires six weeks plaster cast and appropriate physiotherapy support.

Excision arthroplasty

This is often undertaken with synovectomy, commonly at the metatarsal heads, e.g. the Fowler's procedure. However it is also used for distal radial ulnar joint reconstruction where dorsal subluxation of the distal ulnar reduces joint instability as a result of destruction of the triangular cartilage. Excision of the radial head is often used in combination with synovectomy in surgical reconstruction of the elbow to improve joint flexion.

Arthrodesis

Joint fusion is appropriate where the amount of motion required at the joint is relatively limited. Radio-carpal arthrodesis reduces dislocation of the wrist and facilitates fusion in a functional position of 15% to 20% of extension. Fusion of the thumb at the carpo-metacarpal joint is also a beneficial operation, and correction of Boutonniere deformity or instability of the proximal interphalangeal joints of the fingers can improve hand function. Arthrodesis of the shoulder is beneficial if there is significant damage by rheumatoid arthritis or other destructive process. Atalanto-axial subluxation can also be subject of fusion in the cervical spine if more radical surgery is not required.

LOWER LIMB JOINT REPLACEMENT

Total hip replacement

This is the commonest joint replacement undertaken in the Western world, primarily for osteoarthritis patients but is also used frequently for rheumatoid arthritis patients. The commonest form of replacement provides a titanium-femoral component, together with a polyethylene acetabular component. Complete relief of pain occurs in over 90% of rheumatoid arthritis patients and over 95% of patients with Charnley cemented hips are reported to be good or excellent at 15 to 21 year follow-up. The commonest long term problems relate to aseptic loosening, particulate wear resulting from debris from damage to the polyethylene cup and stress bone damage returning from poor bone stock. Revision surgery, when required, is a more extensive operation and the complications of fractures, infections and loosening are more common. Bone grafting is often used to strengthen the supporting bone.

Total knee replacement

Total knee replacement has undergone a series of major design changes to the point that 15 year survival equals that of total hip replacement. The majority of total knee replacements now consist of a metal resurfacing prosthesis applied to the bottom end of the femur with a polyethylene replacement for the tibial plateau (Figure 29.1). Complications include the standard ones following joint replacement but patella subluxation and dislocation of fracture can also occur.

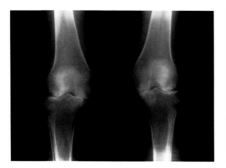 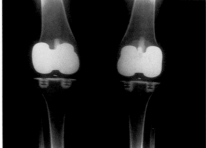

Figure 29.1 *Pre/post operative knee replacement*

Total ankle replacement

This is not commonly undertaken because of the 25% failure rate. Problems occur with rapid loosening but one cause of limited benefit may be because so-called 'ankle pain' can have multiple aetiologies often resulting from destruction and deformity of the hind or fore foot. Ankle arthrodesis provides only limited benefit, but appropriate splinting, locking the tibiotalar ankle joint, prior to surgery can give a clue as to whether arthrodesis would improve symptoms.

UPPER LIMB JOINT REPLACEMENT

Shoulder replacement

Common causes of shoulder pain, such as impingement by synovitis, torn rotator cuff, degenerative disease of the acromio-clavicular joint and pain emanating from the cervical spine, should be excluded prior to arthroplasty.

Pain relief following replacement of the gleno-humoral joint occurs in over 95% of cases. Range and movement can be improved, provided the rotator cuff is intact and functional improvement can allow improved lifestyle in terms of personal hygiene. The commonest replacement consists of a metallic humeral head and a polyethylene glenoid component.

Total replacement of the elbow

Elbow arthroplasty is complicated by the superficial situation of the joint and there is a high incidence of poor wound healing and post-operative sepsis. Instability often occurs as a result of damage to the medial collateral ligaments resulting from the rheumatoid disease process and the ulnar nerve is particularly at risk as it travels round the medial epicondyle. Complications are reported to occur in approximately 25% of cases.

Wrist replacement

This is rarely undertaken because wrist arthrodesis if a more successful operation, but most surgeons are reluctant to fuse both wrists. Bilateral disease is an indication for full wrist replacement. A polyethylene spacer is occasionally inserted within the space usually occupied by the carpus.

Metacarpophalangeal joint replacement

The silastic replacements for the metacarpophalangeal joint improve appearance and pain, but do little for hand function. They often break within ten years of replacement, but newer materials are now being used that fracture less commonly.

Complications of joint replacement

Infection occurs in approximately 1% of patients but is more frequent in those with rheumatoid arthritis. Infection can either occur at the time of surgery, but 15% can occur late due to haematogenous spread, often from rheumatoid ulcers or skin breakdown or infection at other sites. Prophylactic antibiotics should be given for potentially infective procedures such as colonoscopy, urological examination and dental treatment. Presenting symptoms include the usual symptoms of infection together with acute progressively worsening joint pain. If suspected then this is an acute emergency as there is a 15% mortality associated with joint infection. Patients with rheumatoid arthritis are less likely to have a fever or elevated white cell count with joint sepsis.

Infection usually requires prosthesis removal, debridement and consideration for a further replacement three months later. This is not always feasible

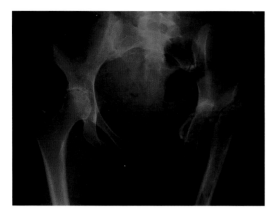

Figure 29.2 *X-ray showing left Girdlestone arthroplasty*

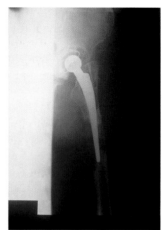

Figure 29.3 *Loose joint replacement*

and occasionally Girdlestone arthroplasty at the hip may be necessary (Figure 29.2). Rarely, amputation may be required in severe cases if medical and surgical options have been exhausted.

Loosening of the replaced joint is manifest by a slower but progressive pain on use of the joint. Joint examination is painful in most modalities and the joint may show laxity of movement. The x-ray shows a lucent line round the prosthetic component (Figure 29.3). Debris from the polyethylene or metal components can be found at the site of the osteolytic lesions implying their involvement in the loosening process. A second replacement may be required.

New bone formation can also occur, particularly in osteoarthritis patients, in up to 40% of cases but it is only clinically troublesome in about 1% to 2%. The pain and stiffness associated with extra-osseous calcification may be helped with analgesics and physiotherapy.

Warning signs of prosthesis loosening include:

- gradual increase in pain;
- instability on joint movement;
- lucent line on x-ray.

SUMMARY

Indications for joint surgery

Surgery is indicated where there is:

- pain;
- instability;
- loss of function.

Warning signs of prosthesis loosening

These include:

- gradual increase in pain;
- instability on joint movement;
- lucent line on x-ray.

Warning signs of infection

These include:

- onset of new pain;
- pain on weight-bearing;
- signs of inflammation;
- site for infection;
- high acute phase response.

Further reading

G. Hosie and J. Dickson, *Managing Osteoarthritis in Primary Care* (Blackwell Science, Oxford, 2000)

J. H. Klippel and P. A. Dieppe, *Rheumatology* (Mosby-Yearbook(Europe) Ltd, London, 1999)

P. Maddison, D. Isenberg, P. Woo and D. Glass, *Oxford Textbook of Rheumatology* (Oxford University Press)

T. Silver, *Joint and Soft Tissue Injections* (2nd edn., Radcliffe Medical Press, Abingdon, 1999)

M. Snaith, *ABC of Rheumatology* (BMJ Publishing Group, London, 1996)

Useful addresses

PRINCIPAL ORGANISATIONS

Arthritis Care
England:
18 Stephenson Way
London NW1 2HD
tel: 020 7916 1500
website: http://www.arthritiscare.org.uk

Scotland:
15 Glasgow Road
Bathgate EH48 2AW
Tel: 01506 631333

Arthritis Research Campaign
Copeman House
St Mary's Gate
Chesterfield S41 7TD
tel: 01246 558033
website: http://www.arc.org.uk

The British Society for Rheumatology
41 Eagle St
London WC1R 4AR
tel: 020 7242 3313
website: http://www.rheumatology.org.uk

Primary Care Rheumatology Society
PO Box 42
Northallerton
North Yorkshire DL7 8YG
tel: 01609 774794

University of Bath and PCR Diploma
University of Bath
Bath BA2 7AY
tel: 01225 826887

FURTHER ORGANISATIONS

Action for Sick Children
(National Association for the Welfare of Children in Hospital)
Argyle House
29-31 Euston Road
London NW1 2SD
tel: 020 8542 4848

British Footwear Association
5 Portland Place
London W1N 3AA
tel: 020 7580 8687

British Sjögren's Syndrome Association
Unit 1
Manor Workshop
West End
Nailsea
Bristol BS19 2DD
website: ourworld.compuserve.com/homepages/bssassociation

Disability Alliance
1st Floor East
Universal House
88-94 Wentworth Street
London E1 7SA
tel: 020 7289 6111
website: http://www.dlf.org.uk

Disablement Information and Advice Line (DIAL UK)
Park Lodge
St Catherine's Hospital
Tickhill Road
Doncaster DN4 8QN
tel: 01302 310123
website: http://members.aol.com.dialuk

Fibromyalgia Association UK
PO Box 206
Stourbridge
PY9 8YL
tel: 01384 820052

Hypermobility Syndrome Association
15 Oakdene
Alton
Hants GU34 2AJ
tel: 01705 345 127
website: http://www.hypermobility.org

Lupus UK
Central James House
Eastern Road
Romford
Essex RM1 3NH
tel: 01708 731251

Mayfield
East Sussex TN20 6ZL
tel: 01435 873527
website: http://web.ukonline.co.uk/nass

National Ankylosing Spondylitis Society
PO Box 179
National Back Pain Association
16 Elmtree Road
Teddington
Middlesex TW11 8ST
tel: 020 8977 5474
website: http://www.backpain.org

National Osteoporosis Society
PO Box 10
Radstock
Bath BA3 3YB
tel: 020 7222 5300
e-mail: l.Edwards@nos.org.uk

Psoriasis Association
Contact: Mrs Johnson
54 Bellevue Road
Edinburgh

Royal Association for Disability and Rehabilitation
12 City Forum
250 City Road
London EC1V 8AF
tel: 020 7250 3222
website: http://www.radar.org.uk

Society of Chiropodists and Podiatrists
1 Fellmongers Path
Tower Bridge Road
London SE1 3LY
tel: 020 7234 8620
website: http://www.feetforlife.org

SPOD (Sexual Problems of the Disabled)
286 Camden Road
London N7 0BJ
tel: 020 7607 8851/2

The Raynaud's & Scleroderma Association
112/114 Crewe Road
Alsager
Cheshire
tel: 01270 872776
website: http://www.raynauds.demon.co.uk

The Scleroderma Society
61 Sandpit Lane
St Albans
Herts
tel: 01727 855054

Index